Springer Series on

REHABILITATION

Volume 1
The Psychology of Disability
Carolyn L. Vash, Ph.D.

Volume 2
Disabled People as Second-Class Citizens
Myron G. Eisenberg, Ph.D., Cynthia Griggins, and Richard J. Duval, Editors

Volume 3
Behavioral Approaches to Rehabilitation: Coping with Change
Elaine Greif, Ph.D. and Ruth G. Matarazzo, Ph.D.

Volume 4
Chronic Illness and Disability through the Life Span: Effects on Self and Family
Myron G. Eisenberg, Ph.D., LaFaye C. Sutkin, Ph.D., and Mary A. Jansen, Ph.D., Editors

Volume 5
Handbook of Private Sector Rehabilitation
Lewis J. Taylor, Ph.D., C.R.C.,
Marjorie Golter, M.S., C.R.C., Gary Golter, M.A., and Thomas E. Backer, Ph.D., Editors

Lewis J. Taylor, Ph.D., a rehabilitation psychologist, has worked as a rehabilitation counselor, trainer, and supervisor in the private sector. A founding partner of American Rehabilitation Management in 1979, he served as its vice-president for operations until 1984. He has taught at the University of Southern California, served as president of NRCA of California, and worked as a rehabilitation psychologist in the Clinical Gerontology Program at Rancho Los Amigos Hospital, a major rehabilitation facility in southern California. He is presently Clinical Services Coordinator for Comprehensive Mental Health Services in Virginia Beach, Virginia.

Marjorie Golter, M.S., is a Certified Rehabilitation Counselor who has worked since 1977 developing computer systems in the area of rehabilitation for both private and public sectors. She is part owner of Rehab Software, a firm whose primary product is VOCOMP, a job-matching system for disabled people. She has also worked as a rehabilitation counselor for a private sector rehabilitation firm. Mrs. Golter completed her master's degree in rehabilitation at the University of Southern California.

Gary Golter, M.A., is part owner and manager of Rehab Software, a computer software firm specializing in the design and marketing of computer-based applications that address the relocation of workers. Prior to 1977, Mr. Golter was a Senior Vice President at Lutheran Hospital Society of Southern California, a nonprofit organization which owns and manages eight hospitals located throughout California. His experience includes positions with Arthur Young & Company, Brokers Data Service, and Technicolor, Inc.

Thomas E. Backer, Ph.D., is senior research scientist, Human Interaction Research Institute; Assistant Research Professor, UCLA School of Medicine; and a consultant in private practice. Dr. Backer has conducted applied research projects for numerous federal human service agencies and is the author of more than 150 books, journal articles, and research reports. He is founding coeditor of the *Annual Review of Rehabilitation* and editor of the Springer Series on Rehabilitation. He is also past-president, Division of Consulting Psychology, American Psychological Association; and Associate Editor, American Psychological Division of Rehabilitation Psychology *Newsletter*.

Handbook of Private Sector Rehabilitation

Lewis J. Taylor, Ph.D., C.R.C.
Marjorie Golter, M.S., C.R.C.
Gary Golter, M.A.
Thomas E. Backer, Ph.D.
Editors

Springer Publishing Company
New York

Springer Publishing Company, Inc.
536 Broadway
New York, New York 10012

85 86 87 88 89 / 10 9 8 7 6 5 4 3 2 1

Library of Congress Cataloging in Publication Data

Main entry under title:
Handbook of private sector rehabilitation.

(Springer series on rehabilitation; v. 5)
Bibliography: p. Includes index.
1. Rehabilitation—United States—Addresses, essays, lectures. I. Taylor, Lewis J. II. Series.
HD7256. U5H36 1985 388.4'73624048'0973 84-26903
ISBN 0-8261-3940-X

Printed in the United States of America

Contents

Contributors

Kerry M. Boyle is President and owner of Comprehensive Rehabilitation Services, Inc. A graduate of San Francisco University, he currently serves on the Board of Directors and as President and Legislative Committee Chair of the California Association of Rehabilitation Professionals.

Peter P. Griswold, M.A., is State Director, Michigan Rehabilitation Services in the Michigan Department of Education. Starting as a counselor in 1956, he is currently President of the Council of State Administrators of Vocational Rehabilitation.

Ronald B. Harper, Ed.D., C.R.C., is President of Ronald B. Harper, Inc., consultants in assessment of employability and vocational rehabilitation. He has been a vocational expert for the Social Security Administration in California and has served as a rehabilitation counselor and supervisor for the California Department of Rehabilitation. Presently a member of the President's Committee on Employment of the Handicapped, he is the recipient of the California Personnel and Guidance Association distinguished service award.

Richard M. Keane, M.Ed., is an associate director with The Travelers Insurance Company and serves as the National Rehabilitation Coordinator. Currently studying for an M.B.A. at the University of Hartford, he is a member of the Connecticut Governor's Committee on Employment of the Handicapped, the Insurance Rehabilitation Study Group, and the National Rehabilitation Association, including the NRCA and Job Placement Divisions.

Jill K. Martin, President of Comprehensive Rehabilitation Services, Inc. of Oregon, has a master of science degree in nursing administration from California State University at Los Angeles. She has been involved in private sector rehabilitation for over eight years in a variety of jobs and responsibilities.

Ralph E. Matkin, Rh.D., C.R.C., serves as a consultant to the Commission on Rehabilitation Counselor Certification and chairs the Task Force on Certification of Rehabilitation Specialists in Insurance. Currently president of Vocational Management Systems, Inc., he is the author of *Voca-*

tional Rehabilitation in an Entrepreneurial System: Challenging New Frontiers, numerous articles, and book chapters.

Shelia S. Newman, M.S., is Senior Research Associate at Planning Systems International, Inc., and has authored several publications on independent living and rehabilitation technology. She has served on research projects of the Rehabilitation Services Administration, the National Institute of Handicapped Research, and the Department of Labor.

Elizabeth L. Pan, Ph.D., is President of Planning Systems International, a consulting and data processing firm. She has served as a project director for a number of studies on the delivery of rehabilitation information and has authored numerous papers and reports on administrative and technical capacities in both the scientific and human services areas.

Debra A. Perry, M.Ed., C.R.C., is a research associate with Planning Systems International, Inc., Falls Church, Virginia. She has worked for Springwood Psychiatric Institute in Leesburg, Virginia, developing and implementing a vocational service program for psychiatric and chemically dependent patients.

Paul Scher, C.R.C., is the Equal Opportunity Manager for the handicapped program at Sears, Roebuck & Company. He presently is involved with the National Affirmative Program and is a consultant to a merchandising organization producing products to help the disabled customer.

Carl E. Shawhan, Ph.D., serves as Director of the National Rehabilitation Job Development/Job Placement Specialist Program at Drake University. He is also a consultant and trainer with private sector organizations and with the business and insurance communities.

Introduction

Lewis J. Taylor, Marjorie Golter, Gary Golter, and Thomas E. Backer

Private sector rehabilitation[1] has come a long way since 1975, when California enacted the first mandatory Workers' Compensation vocational rehabilitation program. Before that, there were only a few rehabilitation practitioners in private practice scattered around the country. Now, according to Ralph Matkin (see Chapter 1), there are more than twice as many new employment opportunities annually for rehabilitation professionals in the private sector as in the public state/federal system. This change is surely the single most significant development in rehabilitation since the rapid growth in the field following World War II.

This new field of private rehabilitation can easily be compared to the old American frontier. There is a hurly-burly atmosphere. People are inventing new ways of providing services and starting new enterprises every day. Competition is keen and the "law" (standard of practice) is developing slowly. For the winners on this frontier, the struggle is exhilarating and the rewards satisfying. But not everyone who stakes a claim to this new territory hangs on to it. Not everyone is well enough prepared—one way or another.

Until 1979, very little had appeared in the rehabilitation literature regarding work in the private sector. Numerous articles have since been published in the professional rehabilitation journals, addressing various private rehabilitation issues. Additionally, a few books have appeared, describing particular state workers' compensation rehabilitation systems. To date, however, there has not been a book published about private sector rehabilitation in all of its major aspects and with a national emphasis. As private rehabilitation spreads across the country and develops many potential applications, rehabilitation professionals will need information about this growing field in order to make career decisions for themselves and to provide better service for their clients. It was to meet this need that we have prepared this volume. Our aim is to show what is going on in private rehabilitation now, where the field has come from, and where it seems to be going. As much

[1]Throughout this volume, the terms "private sector rehabilitation" and "private rehabilitation" will be used interchangeably, both referring to rehabilitation services offered by individuals or profit-making firms for a fee.

as possible, the *Handbook* avoids speaking to any one of the specialist groups such as counselors, evaluators, or job placement specialists. Rather, it invites all rehabilitation professionals to see how they may become involved in this dynamic new professional enterprise.

In the first chapter, Ralph Matkin, Rh.D., describes the present state of rehabilitation in the private sector. He describes the origins of private rehabilitation and the current activities of its practitioners, providing a point of departure for the *Handbook*. Peter Griswold, M.A., State Director of Rehabilitation Services in Michigan, provides in the second chapter an analysis of the relationship between the new private sector and the traditional rehabilitation system. Competition and confrontation between the two systems are described, and the potential for their productive collaboration is suggested. The private sector is the child of traditional rehabilitation, and Griswold reminds us that this relationship should not be ignored.

The next six chapters describe what private sector rehabilitationists are doing today. Richard Keane, M.Ed., National Rehabilitation Coordinator for the Travelers Insurance Company, provides an insider's view of the insurance industry, which is the major source of private rehabilitation referrals. It is not enough, he asserts in his chapter, for the rehabilitation practitioner to have mastered rehabilitation theory and practice—the insurance industry (e.g., its need for and attitudes toward rehabilitation services) must also be understood.

Chapters about providing expert testimony, working as a rehabilitationist in industry, being a consultant, and providing rehabilitation information technology services delineate other areas of private rehabilitation practice. In his chapter, Ronald B. Harper, Ed.D., C.R.C., a rehabilitation consultant in private practice, offers the reader his experience gained as a vocational consultant and expert witness over a more than ten-year period. Dr. Harper describes, in practical terms, what expert vocational testimony is, who does it, and how. Paul Scher, Corporate Manager of the Handicapped Program for Sears Roebuck and Company, describes the utilization of rehabilitation professionals employed by large corporations as part of their human resource development programs. Scher provides extended descriptions of some of the largest in-house rehabilitation programs in private industry.

Many rehabilitationists in the private sector regard themselves as consultants. Thomas E. Backer, Ph.D., a consulting psychologist and past president of the American Psychological Association's Division of Consulting Psychology, offers an overview of the basic principles of organizational consulting as applied to private rehabilitation. Dr. Backer's chapter provides practical information about types of consulting work available to rehabilitationists and describes basic concepts of consulting, training requirements for consultants, and strategies for effective consulting interventions.

The next chapter, by Shelia S. Newman, M.S., Debra Perry, M.Ed., C.R.C., and Elizabeth L. Pan, Ph.D., of Planning Systems International, describes an essential element in private rehabilitation—the injured workers. Newman, Perry, and Pan have assembled information from both published and unpublished sources to describe this client population's unique characteristics. Case studies help the reader understand the factors that may interfere with rehabilitation.

One area of consulting rapidly developing now is the provision of guidance and services in the area of computer applications in rehabilitation. Gary Golter, M.A., general partner in Rehab Software, an information technology consulting firm, describes the use of information technology in private sector rehabilitation. In particular, he describes how information technology is being used by private sector rehabilitation administrators, counselors, and disabled consumers. He provides practical advice on the selection of software, hardware, and consultants, and speculates about the use of computers in rehabilitation in the future.

Many rehabilitation practitioners and graduate students presently outside the private sector are wondering how to "get inside." The next four chapters offer the reader both general concepts and concrete information that can help in this regard. Chapters on professional training, getting started in business as an entrepreneur, marketing rehabilitation services, and planning ahead in business will assist the reader in understanding what it takes to function effectively in the private sector. Carl Shawhan, Ph.D., Director of the National Rehabilitation Job Development/Job Placement Specialist Program at Drake University, leads off this section by describing needs and standards for professional training in private sector rehabilitation. Professor Shawhan's graduate program at Drake illustrates one proven approach to meeting the special training needs of the private sector.

In her chapter, Marjorie Golter, M.S., C.R.C., general partner in Rehab Software and a rehabilitation counselor, describes the nuts and bolts required to put together a small business such as a private rehabilitation firm. Golter reminds us that it is not enough to be a rehabilitation expert. One must also know how to develop a business plan; attract investors; use attorneys, accountants, and banks; design services; hire staff; and order stationery, among many other things. Lack of awareness of these aspects of private practice is probably the main reason for many counselors' failure to maintain successful private practices. Of course, one can do all this well and still go out of business if there is not a sufficient number of referrals or other sources of business every month. In his chapter, Kerry Boyle, President of Comprehensive Rehabilitation Services (California), offers the reader his nearly ten years of rehabilitation marketing experience. The importance of knowing the marketplace, selling services, and providing service after the sale is described clearly in this chapter, and practical advice is given for each of these areas of responsibility.

More than one rehabilitation entrepreneur has been left behind as a result of inadequate planning. Jill K. Martin, President of Comprehensive Rehabilitation Services (Oregon), makes a strong case for considering planning as a vital function of every manager in this dynamic field. In her chapter, Martin describes the need, scope, and process of planning, using examples from private sector rehabilitation drawn from her many years of experience in the field. Planning in areas of finance, facilities, human resources, product development, and marketing are some of the topics she addresses.

The issue of professional ethics is especially important to the private sector as it goes about developing this new frontier of rehabilitation. Lewis J. Taylor, Ph.D., a rehabilitation psychologist, describes the present state of ethics in rehabilitation, identifies the unique characteristics of the private sector that can produce ethical dilemmas for its practitioners, and presents ethical problems and solutions using current ethical guidelines. One of the objectives of this chapter is to encourage the private practitioner to become more aware of ethical issues and to consciously apply professional ethics in his or her daily work.

In our concluding chapter, several issues suggested by one or more of the chapter authors are used to identify future development and implication to be derived from this volume. The interface between rehabilitation and insurance personnel, the objectives of rehabilitation in the private sector, and the difficulties for rehabilitationists becoming entrepreneurs are among these issues.

Much more, of course, can and should be said about the present and future of private sector rehabilitation. We hope that this *Handbook* may stimulate further examination of this relatively new and effective approach to meeting the rehabilitation needs of disabled people.

1 The State of Private Sector Rehabilitation

Ralph E. Matkin

What is private sector rehabilitation? Frequently, the ensuing answer is dependent on whom one asks and that person's frame of reference. Based on a very broad definition of the word "private," it could be said that these are activities designed to serve disabled persons and performed by individuals or agencies which are not publicly controlled. Within this context, private rehabilitation can represent services and activities performed by either not-for-profit private facilities, such as sheltered workshops, or by persons and firms operating in a for-profit capacity. However, the term "private rehabilitation" will be used throughout this chapter to mean those activities performed by or through individuals or agencies in the entrepreneurial business sector. The aim is to provide the reader with information about the state of private rehabilitation and, thus, acquaint him or her with the salient characteristics of this newly emerging area. The chapter is divided into five sections: (1) foundations and philosophy, (2) services and settings, (3) roles and functions of practitioners, (4) qualifications and credentials, and (5) trends and challenges.

Foundations and Philosophy

Between 1920 and 1970, virtually all vocational rehabilitation services were provided by and accomplished through public, tax-supported agencies operating at state and federal levels. This should not be surprising, when one considers that the vocational rehabilitation field was created, shaped, and subsidized primarily by federal mandates and appropriations designed to assist handicapped Americans in returning to work. During this period, the economic and social benefits of restoring handicapped citizens to gainful and productive activities accrued and have been well documented. The successes achieved by vocational rehabilitation services have contributed to the field's growth among allied health service occupations in a short time span. Evidence of federal commitment to the development and expansion of the public vocational rehabilitation program up to the early 1970s was in the form of increased funding for the purposes of (a) providing all necessary services to return handicapped individuals to employment, (b) expanding the number of disability categories eligible to receive services, (c) developing and maintaining rehabilitation counselor training programs in order to prepare more service providers to enter the field, (d) remodeling and constructing additional rehabilitation centers and private not-for-profit facilities to assist the public sector in its service delivery efforts, and (e) encouraging research and demonstration projects to identify ways and means to provide rehabilitation services to handicapped persons not covered to date. On the other hand, passage of the Rehabilitation Act of 1973 marked a turning point for the federally sponsored public program and served to open the door for services to be offered in the private sector.

Service accountability was the hallmark of the 1973 Rehabilitation Act, epitomized by the initiation of an individualized written rehabilitation program for each client and service priority given to those persons with the most severe disabilities. Moreover, by omitting the word "vocational" from the title of the Act, Congress paved the way for the 1978 Amendments to eliminate the long-standing employment feasibility criterion for service eligibility. Thus, the public sector program soon found itself faced with providing services of longer duration and consequently spending more funds per capita in order to habilitate severely disabled clients with very limited or no vocational potential (Matkin, 1983). As a by-product of this modified service delivery focus by state-federal rehabilitation agencies, together with insufficient funding to provide all necessary services to eligible clients, those with less severe disabling conditions began seeking vocational assistance elsewhere.

The growth of private sector vocational rehabilitation also was aided in 1975 when California became the first state to mandate vocational rehabilitation services as part of its workers' compensation statutes. The tendency for insurance carriers and self-insured employers to use the services of private rehabilitation practitioners and firms to assist industrially injured workers to return to employment was based on three factors. First, since the early 1940s insurance companies have been aware of the cost-savings provided by offering prompt vocational rehabilitation services to injured workers employed by their policyholders. Liberty Mutual was the first insurance company to hire rehabilitation nurses to attend to the vocational needs of disabled workers (Lewin, Ramseur, & Sink, 1979). Second, the inflexibility and time-consuming requirements of public rehabilitation agencies decreased case management efficiency and increased service costs (Porter, 1981). Third, the tendency of injured workers was to resist becoming stigmatized by being associated with public assistance programs (Porter, 1981). Finally, growth of private-sector vocational rehabilitation has flourished because of its emphasis on returning disabled persons to employment as expeditiously as possible.

The "return-to-work" philosophy advocated by private vocational rehabilitation service providers generally takes the form of the following hierarchy identified by Matkin (1981) and Welch (1979):

1. Return the client to work performing the same job with the same employer.
2. Return the client to work performing the same (but modified) job with the same employer.
3. Return the client to work performing a different job, capitalizing on transferable skills, with the same employer.
4. Return the client to work performing the same or modified job with a different employer.
5. Return the client to work performing a different job, one that capitalizes on transferable skills, with a different employer.
6. Return the client to work performing a different job, one that requires extensive and prolonged training, with the same or different employer.
7. As a last resort, return the client to work in self-employment.

In reviewing this hierarchy, little difference is noted between public and private sector philosophies of vocational rehabilitation in terms of goals. The similarities are even more apparent when comparing the definitions of rehabilitation provided by the National Council on Rehabilitation and the International Association of International Accident Boards and Commissions (IAIABC):

> The purpose of vocational rehabilitation is the restoration of the handicapped to the fullest physical, mental, social, vocational and economic usefulness of which they are capable. (National Council on Rehabilitation, 1944, p. 6)

> The restoration of an occupationally disabled employee to that person's optimal physical, mental, vocational, and economic usefulness. (IAIABC, 1977, p. 3)

Finally, by returning clients to work in a prompt and effective manner, not only are cost-savings realized in terms of reducing the costs associated with prolonged training programs, but reemployment reduces the anxiety produced by prolonged disruption of family income, while increasing the likelihood of achieving successful vocational placement. Needless to say, this return-to-work philosophy advocated by private sector vocational rehabilitation has a direct bearing on the nature and duration of services offered by the majority of its practitioners.

Services and Settings

Gutowski and his associates (1979, 1980) have indicated that approximately 80% of all services offered in the private vocational rehabilitation sector are directed toward serving workers' compensation claimants, that is, the industrially injured worker. The Office of Workers' Compensation Programs has stated that it considers "private rehabilitation agencies a useful alternative to the public rehabilitation agencies in providing the best and all necessary services to expeditiously return the injured worker to employment" (Department of Labor, 1980, p. 1). In order to meet the challenge of returning disabled clients to employment as soon as is medically feasible, services offered by private rehabilitation practitioners tend to be placement-oriented, short-term in duration, and vocational in nature (McMahon, 1979; Scher, 1979). This claim was substantiated by Matkin's (1982) research into the roles and functions of rehabilitation specialists working in the private sector. Among the 29 service areas identified in that study, the first 11 are listed in Table 1–1 along with the percentage of members of the National Association of Rehabilitation Professionals in the Private Sector (NARPPS) offering them.

It is apparent from the percentage of private rehabilitation specialists providing the services listed in Table 1–1 that a dramatic division occurs be-

Table 1–1. Services Offered among NARPPS Members

Services	*Percent*
1. Vocational counseling	94.8
2. Job analysis	92.0
3. Job placement	90.8
4. Job development	88.5
5. Case monitoring and follow-up	86.8
6. Labor market surveying	84.5
7. Vocational evaluation	76.4
8. Medical case management	76.4
9. Vocational testimony	71.3
10. Job restructuring consultation	70.1
11. Psychological evaluation	40.8

tween the tenth most frequently offered service (job restructuring consultation) and the eleventh (psychological evaluation). Among those services even less frequently offered are psychological counseling (40.2%), work adjustment (35.6%), independent living skills training (20.1%), and job-seeking skills training (5.2%), each of which receives much greater emphasis in public sector rehabilitation programs (Matkin, 1982). Keeping in mind the private sector's return-to-work orientation, as well as the high incidence of workers' compensation caseload composition, it is quite understandable that long-term treatment programs are minimally provided. Similarly, from a workers' compensation framework, it can be assumed that the presence of a work history among claimants further reduces the necessity for such services as job-seeking skills, independent living training, and work adjustment counseling in the private sector. More importantly, however, the services identified in Table 1–1 are offered in most private rehabilitation work settings.

Since the inception of the state-federal vocational rehabilitation program, preparation of rehabilitation professionals, especially counselors, has focused on their ultimate employment in the public sector. In the mid-1970s it was estimated that 50% of the approximately 20,000 rehabilitation counselors nationwide worked in state agencies (Schumacher, 1977). More recently, reduced federal appropriations to public rehabilitation programs and a depressed economic climate have resulted in a decreasing demand for professional manpower in the traditional rehabilitation workplace (Geist & McMahon, 1981). On the other hand, employment opportunities for rehabilitation counselors, vocational evaluators, and job placement specialists have been projected as increasing in private rehabilitation work settings through 1983 (Gutowski, 1979; Gutowski et al., 1980; McFarlane & DiPaola, 1979). Furthermore, while the private sector accounted for approximately 10% of the total employment of counselors in 1978, the net changes in counseling and placement positions available in the private sector ranged from 23% in 1979 to 31% by 1983 (Gutowski, 1979). Indeed, the study of employment trends in the rehabilitation field that was conducted by the Urban Institute projected that by 1983 twice as many employment opportunities would exist in the private sector compared to the state-federal vocational rehabilitation system (Gutowski, 1979).

As mentioned earlier, private rehabilitation is the term used to define activities performed for disabled persons by profit-making business enterprises. The most frequently offered services by this sector have been identified. At this point, more specific definition is required regarding the types of business settings where private rehabilitation professionals are employed. Among the assorted businesses subsumed by private rehabilitation are such entities as corporations in any industry, rehabilitation companies, insurance companies, large law firms, private hospitals, nursing homes, and private practitioners (Hasbrook, 1981). During a recent investigation of the National

Association of Rehabilitation Professionals in the Private Sector (NARPPS) membership, Matkin (1982) reported that more than half of the respondents (55.1%) were self-employed rehabilitation specialists who either employed other rehabilitation specialists (40.2%) or worked independently (14.9%). Table 1–2 has been constructed to provide additional information about the nature and types of employment settings where private vocational rehabilitation specialists are working.

In addition to learning the types of services offered and the nature of the employment settings among members of NARPPS, Matkin (1982) discovered that approximately 5,300 personnel were currently serving in a vocational rehabilitation capacity in over 1,200 offices nationwide in the private sector. Because of the magnitude of these numbers, it is understandable that information would be necessary about the work characteristics of these persons. A work role delineation study, concentrating on rehabilitation specialists in the private sector, would provide useful information about the potential training needs of these practitioners, as well as providing guidelines to colleges and universities responsible for their initial preparation in the field of vocational rehabilitation.

Roles and Functions of Practitioners

Establishment of rehabilitation counselor educational programs and the creation of more job openings for rehabilitation graduates were two of the principal hallmarks of the 1954 Vocational Rehabilitation Act Amendments (P.L. 83–565). Clearly this piece of federal legislation was responsible for the subsequent establishment and expansion of training curricula to meet the needs of practicing rehabilitation counselors in terms of employment preparation. Furthermore, this expanded emphasis directed toward practitioner preparation prior to job entry in the state-federal vocational rehabilitation agency system prompted research investigations to identify the work roles and functions of counselors within that system. Studies, such as those performed by Muthard and Salomone (1969) and Wright and Fraser (1975), have served to shape the existing curriculum, accreditation, and certification standards for the field of rehabilitation counseling. Notwithstanding their respective contributions to the field, however, these studies are more applicable to work in the public rehabilitation sector than they are to the private arena. This deficit in private sector content resulted from the simple fact that few persons provided vocational rehabilitation services outside of the state-federal system until the latter part of the 1970s. Since that time, though, various authors have indicated a need to revise the rehabilitation counselor content curriculum to include training in such areas as labor market forecasting, job analysis, job modification, job development and place-

Table 1–2. Employment Settings Among NARPPS Members

Employment Setting	*Percent*
1. Self-employed owner/co-owner with rehabilitation members	40.2
2. Employee of a private vocational rehabilitation company	20.7
3. Employee of an insurance company	17.8
4. Self-employed rehabilitation specialist without other rehabilitation employees	14.9
5. Employee of a nonprofit rehabilitation facility	2.3
6. Employee of a self-insured business	1.7
7. Other	2.3

ment, medical case management, vocational testimony, business marketing, and labor-management relations (Matkin, 1980; McMahon, 1979; Sales, 1979).

The most frequently provided service areas listed in Table 1–1 tend to support the need for curriculum revision and/or modification for persons wishing to enter private sector vocational rehabilitation work. Indeed, Matkin's (1982) research of the roles and functions of private sector rehabilitation practitioners identified five major and 15 minor categories of work activities from his Rehabilitation Specialist Task Inventory (see Table 1–3). As one would expect, on the other hand, the importance attributed to these various job activities is dependent on who performs them (e.g., rehabilitation counselor, nurse, or administrator) and the nature of the employment setting. In the latter instance, Matkin and Rubin and their associates (Matkin et al., 1982; Rubin et al., in press) investigated the effects of the employment on the work functions of Certified Rehabilitation Counselors (C.R.C.) and rehabilitation administrators.

Rehabilitation Counselors

Rehabilitation counselors working in the private sector, who are graduates of accredited graduate training programs in rehabilitation or C.R.C.s, indicate that their major job responsibilities involve case management (i.e.,

Table 1–3. Roles and Functions of Private Sector Rehabilitation Specialists

Major Work Categories and Subcategories
I. Planning and Coordinating Client Services
A. Client orientation and service planning
B. Resource identification and referral
C. Service coordinating
D. Gathering and synthesizing information
E. Guidance and counseling
F. Dissemination of information
II. Business and Office Management
A. Program planning and evaluation
B. Supervisory management
C. Fiscal management
D. Professional growth
III. Job Development and Placement
A. Vocational counseling
B. Job-seeking services
C. Employment negotiation
D. Labor market analysis
E. Job modification
IV. Diagnostic Assessment
V. Other Professional Activities

planning and coordinating client services), job development and placement, and diagnostic assessment (interpretation and integration of evaluation results rather than administration and scoring assessment measures). These findings are true for vocational rehabilitation counselors regardless of whether they were employed by private rehabilitation companies or worked in private practice. On the other hand, business and office management duties were performed either by rehabilitation administrators or else by rehabilitation counselors only if they were involved in private practice.

Rehabilitation Nurses

Despite the fact that rehabilitation nurses have been involved in private sector rehabilitation longer than any other vocationally oriented occupational group, little has been written about their contributions to the field in this capacity. Matkin's (1982) study revealed that nurses perceive their role in the vocational process to be primarily that of service planner and coordinator. In fact, their valuation of that functional capacity exceeded all other groups of private rehabilitation service providers in terms of relative importance to other functional categories. Generally speaking, rehabilitation nurses tend to become involved with injured clients soon after a disability has been sustained, much earlier than rehabilitation counselors. This is an extremely important period for rehabilitation intervention because it allows the professional the opportunity to become part of the treatment team at the onset and offers psychological reassurance to clients that their vocational needs are integrally related to their medical rehabilitation treatment program.

Rehabilitation Administrators

Although not directly involved in research applicable to private sector rehabilitation work roles and functions, this group of rehabilitation personnel were studied in a separate investigation performed by Matkin, Sawyer, Lorenz, and Rubin (1982). From that study, conducted among rehabilitation administrators and supervisors employed in public agencies and not-for-profit rehabilitation facilities, several generalities can be made for those working in the private sector. The validity of the conclusions drawn from the job responsibilities of administrators working in nonprofit facilities for their counterparts in the private sector rests on the fact that in both cases these personnel are concerned with creating a profit for their respective employers. Therefore, the only real difference between these settings has to do with how and to whom the profits are distributed; to the stockholders (i.e., for-profit business) or to be reinvested in the company (i.e., not-for-profit). Rehabilitation administrators in private rehabilitation perform such activities as a normal part of their jobs, which include general management of personnel and professional staff, fiscal management, program planning and evaluation, public relations, and marketing services. On the other hand, the smaller the business in terms of staff size, the more often rehabilitation administrators also have to perform direct service to clients, such as counseling and case management.

Based upon the roles and functions identified in Table 1–3 among private rehabilitation professionals and the subsequent overview of their responsibilities, it is apparent that overlapping duties occur among practitioners who come to their positions with various and assorted background training. Scher (1979) and others have indicated that private rehabilitation service providers have diverse educational and experiential backgrounds despite performing many of the same duties. For example, among the many specialty areas represented by those calling themselves "rehabilitation specialists" are business administration, psychology, social work, insurance claims adjusting, teaching, law, and vocational guidance and counseling, not to mention credentialed rehabilitation counselors, rehabilitation nurses, rehabilitation educators, rehabilitation administrators, vocational evaluators, and work adjustment specialists to name only a few. In view of this diversely trained group of private rehabilitation specialists, it seems important to briefly discuss professional training and credentials necessary for this type of work.

Qualifications and Credentials

It has been reported that well over half (61%) of the persons currently practicing in the private rehabilitation sector have at least a master's degree, approximately 37% are C.R.C.s and 25% are registered nurses, 71% have between one and five years work experience in the private sector, and over half (56%) handle caseloads of 11 to 30 clients per month (Matkin, 1982). For those persons who have graduated from accredited rehabilitation counselor training programs, the knowledge and skills they possess typically are grounded in educational curricula that has remained basically unchanged since the mid-1950s. Programs in rehabilitation were founded on clinical or counseling psychology, or vocational guidance knowledge bases. Current information suggests that these emphases provide firm foundations of knowledge and primary counseling skills but are not focused enough to meet the needs of private rehabilitation professionals, particularly those working within a workers' compensation framework.

Research into the training needs of practicing rehabilitation professionals in the private sector has suggested that the ten most critical areas of knowledge and skill for practice are, in order of importance, (1) functional limitations of disability, (2) employability and transferable skill assessment, (3) job placement and job-seeking skills techniques, (4) rehabilitation planning, (5) workers' compensation legislation, (6) professional ethics, (7) interpersonal communication skills, (8) writing skills, (9) job analysis and job modification, and (10) job-development techniques (Lynch & Martin, 1982). These findings, along with previously mentioned studies, prompted separate reports from NARPPS and the National Council on Rehabilitation Education (NCRE) addressing the need for curriculum revision of rehabilitation counselor education programs accredited by the Council on Rehabilitation Education. Despite the independence of these two reports, their conclusions were strikingly similar as is evident in their recommendations for curriculum modification as summarized below (McMahon & Matkin, in press):

1. Full scope of private sector settings and activities beyond rehabilitation of the industrially injured worker.

2. Workers' compensation issues, such as history and philosophy, insurance matters in the rehabilitation process, claims handling, and the special needs of self-insured employers.
3. Program planning and evaluation methodologies.
4. Medical case management as related and contrasted to vocational management and medical/psychosocial aspects of disability.
5. Case management, service coordination, and follow-up.
6. Vocational evaluation methods.
7. Gathering, synthesizing, and reporting information to different audiences.
8. Identification and utilization of short-term vocational training programs, including assessment of labor market trends, job analysis, and job modification and restructuring.
9. Casefinding methods and techniques for private sector rehabilitation.
10. Legal and ethical issues, such as vocational expert testimony, malpractice issues, privacy and confidentiality, and credentialing.
11. Electives, such as business or rehabilitation administration, fiscal management and budgeting, and employee selection and supervision.

Appropriate training in the occupational discipline is an extremely important factor in the assessment of the qualifications of any service provider. For example, if rehabilitation counseling is to be provided, the consumer most likely would seek a person trained in that field to provide services. The same goes for consumers or employers seeking the services of nurses, physicians, employment counselors, and so on. In the rehabilitation field, however, few regulations exist to protect the welfare of consumers seeking vocational rehabilitation services. Only six states thus far require rehabilitation counselors to be licensed in order to practice (i.e., Alabama, Arkansas, Florida, Idaho, Texas, and Virginia). On the other hand, licensure bills were before the legislatures of approximately 26 states in 1983. For the time being, however, certification and registration are the two principal methods of credentialing rehabilitation service providers.

Certification is available to rehabilitation counselors in the form of the C.R.C. (Certified Rehabilitation Counselor), which is issued by the Commission on Rehabilitation Counselor Certification. Recently, vocational evaluators and work adjustment specialists began their own certification process through the Commission on Certification of Work Adjustment and Vocational Evaluation Specialists (CCWAVES). These bodies represent nongovernmental agencies designed to set minimum acceptable standards of knowledge and skills covering their respective disciplines. Moreover, certification by these agencies means that there is a form of title-control over the use of these disciplinary titles. Title-control also occurs in the form of credentialing known as registration. In the rehabilitation field, several registries exist which include Registered Rehabilitation Therapist, Registered Rehabilitation Specialist, National Certified Counselor, and Registered Nurse, to name a few. As with other forms of credentials, possession of these titles is restricted to those persons who have demonstrated knowledge and skills applicable to their respective disciplines by meeting formal training requirements and examination criteria. Moreover, depending on accompanying state statutes pertaining to these occupations and their services, restraint of practice may be included. More specifically, where state laws exist that indicate a requirement for a registration or certification to be possessed, not only is the occupational title in question controlled, but more importantly, the activities of the occupation(s) are restricted to those possessing the controlled title. In many respects, this type of regulation is akin to licensure because of its strict nature. Thus, as the field of rehabilitation continues to professionally mature, it is conceivable that increased regulations will be imposed in order to further protect the welfare of consumers.

Trends and Challenges

The area of private sector vocational rehabilitation is perhaps one of the fastest growing employment settings in all of the allied health care professions. Along with that growth, though, are associated problems that will require prompt attention and acceptable resolution. Among the areas already mentioned that will present the greatest challenges are adequate preservice and inservice training and credentialing of service providers. In many respects, however, these extremely important issues are at this moment being dealt with by such groups as NARPPS, NCRE, Council on Rehabilitation Education, National Rehabilitation Counseling Association, American Rehabilitation Counseling Association, Job Placement Division, National Employment Counselor Association, Vocational Evaluation and Work Adjustment Association, and the Rehabilitation Insurance Nursing Group. Furthermore, steps are being taken by the Commission on Rehabilitation Counselor Certification to develop and field test a certification examination for rehabilitation specialists in insurance. This effort is particularly noteworthy because of its interdisciplinary approach and scope.

The years to come will reveal how dynamic the field of vocational rehabilitation is, and how it will thoroughly permeate heretofore unseen realms. The challenge before each of us is twofold: we must continue to upgrade our individual skills and those of our respective disciplines, and we must persist in our efforts to consolidate our collective human service skills in order to demonstrate to others the merits of rehabilitation regardless of our employment settings.

References

Department of Labor, Employment Standards Administration. *Guidelines for rehabilitation services from private rehabilitation agencies*. Washington, D.C.: Author, 1980.

Geist, G. O., & McMahon, B. T. Pre-service rehabilitation education: Where graduates are employed. *Journal of Rehabilitation*, 1981, *47*(3), 45–47.

Gutowski, M. *Rehabilitation in the private sector: Changing the structure of the rehabilitation industry*. Washington, D.C.: The Urban Institute, 1979.

Gutowski, M., Harder, P., & Koshel, J. *Forecasting manpower needs in the private rehabilitation industry*. Washington, D.C.: The Urban Institute, 1980.

Hasbrook, R. F. If you have it—Flaunt it. *Journal of Applied Rehabilitation Counseling*, 1981, *12*, 143-145.

International Association of Industrial Accident Boards and Commissions. *Model medical care and rehabilitation program*. Atlanta: Author, 1977.

Lewin, S. S., Ramseur, J. H., & Sink, J. M. The role of private rehabilitation: Founder, catalyst, competitor. *Journal of Rehabilitation*, 1979, *45*(3), 16–19.

Lynch, R. K., & Martin, T. Rehabilitation counseling in the private sector: A training needs survey. *Journal of Rehabilitation*, 1982, *48*(3), 51–53, 73.

Matkin, R. E. The rehabilitation counselor in private practice: Perspectives for education and preparation. *Journal of Rehabilitation*, 1980, *46*(2), 60–62.

Matkin, R. E. Program evaluation: Searching for accountability in private rehabilitation. *Journal of Rehabilitation*, 1981, *47*(1), 65–68.

Matkin, R. E. The roles and functions of rehabilitation specialists in the private sector. (Doctoral dissertation, Southern Illinois University, Carbondale, 1982). *Dissertation Abstracts International*, 1982, *43*, 05A.

Matkin, R. E. Rehabilitation services in the private sector—An expanding area. In S. E. Rubin & R. T. Roessler, (Eds.), *Foundations of the vocational rehabilitation process* (2nd ed.). Baltimore: University Park Press, 1983.

Matkin, R. E., Sawyer, H. W., Lorenz, J. R., & Rubin, S. E. Rehabilitation administrators and supervisors: Their work assignments, training needs, and suggestions for preparation. *Journal of Rehabilitation Administration*, 1982, *6*, 170–183.

McFarlane, F. R., & DiPaola, S. M. Rehabilitation counselor, vocational evaluator and work adjustment specialist: Are these professions different? *Journal of Applied Rehabilitation Counseling*, 1979, *10*, 148–153.

McMahon, B. T. Private sector rehabilitation: Benefits, dangers, and implications for preparation. *Journal of Rehabilitation*, 1979, *45*(3), 56–58.

McMahon, B. T., & Matkin, R. E. Preservice graduate training for private sector rehabilitation counselors: NCRE and NARPPS task force investigations. *Rehabilitation Counseling Bulletin*, in press.

Muthard, J. E., & Salomone, P. R. Roles and functions of the rehabilitation counselor. *Rehabilitation Counseling Bulletin*, 1969, *13*, 81–168.

National Council on Rehabilitation. *Symposium on the process of rehabilitation*. Cleveland: Author, 1944.

Porter, T. L. Foreword. In L. J. Deneen & T. A. Hessellund, *Vocational rehabilitation of the injured worker*. San Francisco: Rehab Publications, 1981.

Rubin, S. E., Matkin, R. E., Ashley, J. M., Beardsley, M. M., May, V. R., Onstott, K. L., & Puckett, F. The roles and functions of certified rehabilitation counselors. *Rehabilitation Counseling Bulletin*, in press.

Sales, A. Rehabilitation counseling in the private sector: Implications for graduate education. *Journal of Rehabilitation*, 1979, *45*(3), 59–61, 72.

Scher, P. L. NARPPS — Key to the survival of rehabilitation in the nineteen-eighties. *Journal of Rehabilitation*, 1979, *45*(3), 50–51, 74.

Schumacher, B. Rehabilitation counseling. In P. J. Valletutti & F. Christoplos (Eds.), *Interdisciplinary approaches to human services*. Baltimore: University Park Press, 1977.

Welch, G. T. The relationship of rehabilitation with industry. *Journal of Rehabilitation*, 1979, *45*(3), 24–25.

Wright, G. N., & Fraser, R. T. Task analysis for the evaluation, preparation, classification and utilization of rehabilitation counselor-track personnel. *Wisconsin Studies in Rehabilitation* (Monograph of the Rehabilitation Research Institute), Madison: University of Wisconsin, 1975, *3*(22).

2 The Relationship of Private Sector Rehabilitation to Traditional Rehabilitation Systems

Peter P. Griswold

Vocational rehabilitation services in America can be divided into three different efforts: a) private nonprofit, b) public, c) private-for-profit.[1] These are listed in their order of origin. These efforts are not isolated, however, as vocational rehabilitation has been administered by these groups not only singly but in combination.

The purpose of this chapter is to review the emergence of private-for-profit rehabilitation agencies and their relationship to state rehabilitation agencies (public) from the perspective of a state agency director. Of special concern is the as yet untapped potential and promise in the collaboration between the state vocational rehabilitation agency and the private-for-profit rehabilitation company.

As might be expected when potential competition emerges, there has been a general concern over the growth of private agencies on the part of state agencies. This concern might well be misplaced if state agencies accept as their mission the expansion and improvement of vocational rehabilitation services to individuals with disabilities through the utilization of all available resources, private as well as public. When, as Dr. Frank Bowe pointed out, "By the year 2000, there will be one chronically ill, over sixty-five or disabled citizen for every able-bodied citizen in this country" (1980), we might well encourage the development of private sector rehabilitation to assist the public effort.

Despite Dr. Bowe's contention (1980) that the public's cost of not rehabilitating its citizens may exceed $150 billion per year in related mainte-

[1]Although state agencies have a variety of designations, for the purposes of this article the State Vocational Rehabilitation agency is abbreviated "SVR," while the private-for-profit agencies are abbreviated "PFP."

nance, health care, and income transfer for costs, public financial support for rehabilitation has continually fallen short of meeting this projected need. The public has not recognized the economic implications of its failure to fully support rehabilitation services for its disabled and often dependent citizens. A more enlightened view and a model for public agencies to emulate has been the effort of business and industry to implement corporate policies to rehabilitate the disabled worker. This effort is recognized as not only humanitarian and good personnel practice, but one that is cost effective. Although a number of companies established such rehabilitation programs voluntarily prior to workers' compensation legislation, it was the advent of these laws mandating rehabilitation that gave rise in many states to private-for-profit rehabilitation service companies. California, Michigan, and Georgia are prime examples of the rapid growth of these PFP companies in response to such legislation.

This development is typical of the maturation and public acceptance of social programs. First, there is a private charitable response to a social concern. Second, public support encourages social legislation. Third, service is mandated by the liability of private organizations. And finally, private citizens purchase services based on the commonly recognized worth of the services. The last stage is not yet well developed in this country in rehabilitation, but it is an inevitable development that will stimulate public and private efforts to address citizens' needs.

Critical Differences between SVR and PFP Agencies

The most significant difference between public and PFP sectors lies in the type of clients each group currently serves. These distinctions in clientele derive from the unique objectives of each sector. PFPs were developed to serve companies that were liable for the rehabilitation of industrially injured workers without regard to the degree of severity of the disability. In actual practice, many of the most severely disabled workers were not feasible for long-term vocational rehabilitation and were offered cash redemption as compensation. PFPs, typically, serve individuals who have had a history of employment. Most companies wish to reemploy their disabled workers to avoid high compensation costs as well as to demonstrate corporate concern for their work force. Thus, the PFPs have had both a clientele with a work history and a likely preestablished vocational placement strategy. Contrasted with this is the public mandate to SVRs to serve all eligible handicapped citizens, a mandate which broadens the range to include, for example, the developmentally disabled persons who usually have had neither employment histories nor established vocational solutions. Public agencies are also under a mandate to serve severely disabled individuals as a priority, so that their problem solution activity may be long-range and more expensive.

A second difference is in-service philosophy. According to George Welch, PFPs have these objectives in order of performance for their clients (Welch, 1979):

1. Return to work in the same job and the same employer.
2. Return to work in a different job and the same employer.
3. Return to work in a different job and a different employer.

Notable is that all three efforts address returning to work, while as indicated earlier, SVRs deal with a large percentage of clients who have never worked. Consequently, service philosophy and program must differ.

The most obvious difference between SVR and PFP agencies is, of course, their respective sources of income. For the SVR it is the public treasury. For the PFP it is the private person and public or private institutions.

In summary, the three major points of difference between SVR and PFP agencies lie in the funding base, the type of client, and the service solutions.

Competition and Confrontation

The early relationship between PFPs and SVRs has been characterized by competition and confrontation on a number of fronts. As private agencies proliferated, their public utterances often contained exaggerated critical evaluations of SVR agencies. It appeared that they were justifying their existence by a denigration of the public effort. Perhaps the constant barrage of criticism was expected to motivate insurance companies and other privately funded programs to refer clients to PFPs rather than to SVRs. This approach can be characterized by the apocryphal story of the disabled truck driver whose rehabilitation plan proposed by the state agency included a six-year college program. This oft-repeated story usually brought derisive laughs from the speaker's audience and pointed out the follies of public efforts while reserving professional competence for the private effort. At the same time, SVRs were castigating PFPs as working for the employer to the possible disadvantage of the client.

Telling of such stories may be natural for competing groups, but they do little to advance the larger cause of rehabilitation. If Frank Bowe contends that there is too little understanding of vocational rehabilitation among the population at large, internal destructive criticism can do little to develop public support. Indeed one of the purposes of this chapter and of previous efforts (e.g., Griswold & Scott, 1979) is to encourage the establishment of a common ground between these sectors for mutual assistance in public education about and promotion of vocational rehabilitation.

There are some advantages to healthy competition, however. The first is the obvious outcome of most competitive ventures—the drive to produce a product superior to that of your competitor. As private agencies have worked to outperform the more established public services, the SVRs in turn have moved to correct their performance inadequacies. PFP companies claim an ability to work with clients without the encumbrances of state/federal regulations that may limit the scope of service and that often result in a slower response to client needs. State agencies, particularly in those states where PFPs are expanding, have paid special attention to alert, responsive service to demonstrate their capability to move as quickly and effectively as PFPs. In this case, PFPs have served as healthy competition. On the other hand, state agencies have played a leading role in accountability and overall productivity. PFPs are now moving in the direction that many SVRs took years ago—equating outputs with resources and holding staff accountable for client success.

As profit is the driving force for private agencies, high productivity is necessary for survival, and SVR staff who have transferred to PFPs are learning to accept that reality. PFPs are developing their own "red tape" and management control systems.

Competition has taken an unhealthy turn, however, in the area of referral sources and qualified staff. The main arena for referral sources has been in the insurance field, especially workers' compensation. States vary in their approach to this type of insurance, and some examples might illustrate these differences.

California, for example, mandated in 1976 rehabilitation provisions within its workers' compensation law and thus provided an early and fertile ground for the establishment of private agencies. The state maintains a compensation unit but serves only about 5% of the state's workers' compensation caseload. Ohio is atypical of other states in the establishment of an Industrial Commission that handles both the compensation and rehabilitation services under the aegis of the state. This is therefore an area where private rehabilitation has gained no strong foothold.

Georgia and Michigan have a larger proportion of compensation cases served by the state rehabilitation agency than by private agencies. Georgia's SVR currently serves 87%, while Michigan's serves 65%. Michigan and Georgia coordinate their programs through their workers' compensation bureaus, with referrals to either the public or a private agency at the option of the insurance carrier. The disabled individual has little protection or choice in the referral, but a handicapped citizen has legal access to the public program as do all other disabled individuals in the state. Occasionally this allows a dual referral, but most often, rehabilitation clients who have been unsuccessful in private efforts will gravitate to the public agency through welfare or health agency referral.

Private agencies spend more time than public agencies do in cultivating referral sources through aggressive marketing, as their motivation is different. In Michigan, for example, about one in ten potentially eligible persons is served by the SVR agency, and counselor caseloads exceed the federal standard of 85 by 50%. There is little motivation to further stimulate referrals when current caseloads are already excessive. PFPs, conversely, are in need of a steady flow of referrals to survive financially.

Another area that brings concern to both groups, but more particularly to the state agencies, is personnel recruitment and retention. For the past decade the vast majority of PFP staff have come from SVR agencies. In Michigan alone, six private companies have been founded by former state agency employees. California and Georgia (Diamond & Petkas, 1979) have experienced the same development.

Once established, many private companies recruit other public rehabilitation counselors by offering a higher salary and an "easier" job that is relatively free from the paperwork and restrictions of public service. By choosing only the most experienced counselors with established referral networks and reputations, the private agency may critically drain the state agencies of talented staff. While this is a reality in any area of work, it does place the public agency in the position of absorbing preservice and in-service training costs, only to lose employees to private agencies who do not have to invest in these high staff development costs.

PFP agencies are to be credited, nevertheless, for their leadership in seeking high credentials for professional staff (Scher, 1979). The motivation here is to portray to insurance companies and the self-insured referral sources that their staffs are professional. State agencies fall considerably behind this effort as they may have constricting personnel practices within their jurisdiction. Georgia, in recognition of this development, has developed strict credentials required for rehabilitation counselors working with workers' compensation clients.

Competition has taken another tack that creates a dilemma for some state agencies. PFP organizations in those states with mandated rehabilitation provisions in their workers' compensation laws have consistently requested that public agencies charge administrative overhead costs. Michigan provides an example of this situation, as a state statute was recently passed to permit the charge back of administrative costs to insurance agencies referring workers' compensation clients for service (Michigan Public Act 315). The direct service cost of the individual client's rehabilitation program had been previously borne by the insurance company, but the administration, counseling, and placement costs were borne by the state's general fund. PFP agencies now wish other states to charge back such costs because, from their perspective, the current situation in states without legislation as exists in Michigan gives an unfair economic advantage for the SVR agency. Their arguments to the state legislature, therefore, are couched in terms that address the cost containment potential for state government, the appeal to full utilization of similar benefits, and the rights of free enterprise. California is another state that does charge administrative overhead and, in the author's judgment, finds no particular disadvantage in doing so. It would seem also that states which could recapture these costs would mount more aggressive workers' compensation programs, placing them in further competition and potential conflict with PFPs.

A Survey in Michigan

In order to review the current relationships between state agencies and private rehabilitation agencies, a survey was conducted in Michigan of 20 PFP rehabilitation companies. In addition, interviews were conducted with Georgia and California state agency representatives who had a primary responsibility for establishing and maintaining relationships with the private sector. The PFP companies are characterized as very small (under 10 staff) and were established within the past ten years.

In the Michigan survey of 20 PFP agencies, 12 agencies responded by mail, 9 stating they had a current working agreement or relationship with Michigan Rehabilitation Services (the SVR agency). The nature of this agreement in six cases was an informal arrangement, with only one organization stating it had a formal written agreement. Five agencies described their major work as that of making referrals to the state agency for services, two stated there was mutual planning and shared service responsibility between the agencies with their clients, while three received referrals from state agencies for psychological testing. One agency received referrals for vocational assessment and one for counseling services. There were no referrals from the state agency to a private company for training or placement services. The survey findings are presented briefly below.

There was a virtual split in response to the question of whether there was a free exchange of client information within the scope of client confidentiality constraints. Five agencies responded that there was a free exchange, four stated that there was not, and one agency qualified its response by saying in some cases there was and in some cases there was not free exchange.

Each company was asked to characterize their relationship to Michigan Rehabilitation Services on a five-point scale ranging from highly cooperative (1) to adversarial (5). This resulted in an almost perfect bell shaped curve with a distribution of 2–2–5–2–1. Eleven agencies wished to improve the relationship, and one did not.

When the agencies were asked to recommend improvements, the following responses were given:

1. With regard to referrals from SVR to PFP, four respondents declared that a referral process was needed.
2. Michigan SVR agency counselors should be trained in workers' compensation and no-fault legislation; two respondents felt that many state agency counselors had limited understanding of these fields.
3. Copies of psychological tests and medical reports should be available from the state agency; one request for this type of cooperation was made.
4. Education for SVR counselors to clarify that private agencies had an equal concern for their clients and that ethical practice and client advocacy were not the sole province of the state agency; one recommendation of this nature was given.
5. Mutual case planning between the agencies with shared responsibility for client outcome was advocated; one recommendation that encouraged such a joint effort was made.

The survey suggests that a large number of Michigan PFP agencies have working agreements or relationships established in their communities with the SVR agency. Most private agencies have geographical limitations, and this difference may limit them more on their location than on their ability to forge good working arrangements with the state. The variety of the nature of these arrangements is reflected in the widespread services that agencies provide, although the survey revealed no referrals for placement services and documented an equal distribution of referrals from private to public and from public to private.

The survey responses on client confidentiality would suggest the need for more formal working arrangements, a mutual understanding of the legal constraints on confidentiality, and the need for enhancing client participation in the process.

The survey responses indicate that the private agencies feel there is a cooperative and acceptable relationship, and even the one adversarial response was addressed more to the political arena than to the service relationship. It is not surprising that the vast majority wish to improve the PFP-SVR relationship. It should be noted that the one PFP agency that did not desire improvement is a company that already enjoys a highly cooperative arrangement with the SVR.

It was somewhat surprising that there was a paucity of specific responses as to how to improve the PFP-SVR relationship, but perhaps the nature of the questionnaire did not encourage such elaboration. Only one respondent wrote a separate letter outlining a number of areas of possible expansion. Most popular was the obvious need for referrals from the state to the private sector. The one comment on the state's need to apprise its counselors that private agencies have an equal and abiding concern for the welfare of clients harkens back to the developmental history of mistrust between SVRs and PFPs. The fact that this concern surfaced only once suggests that much progress has already been made.

The Development of Collaborative Arrangements

There is a need to develop a strong collaborative relationship between private and public agencies, paralleling the longstanding relationship between public and private nonprofit agencies. The problems of disablement and disadvantage are so pervasive in our society that mobilization of our nation's available resources is essential. The long history of nonprofit rehabilitation is rich with success. The public program has evolved to be a comprehensive solution to the employment problems of handicapped persons, its success limited by constrained resources. A logical development would be to forge a strong partnership between these sectors to respond to the growing social recognition of the benefits of rehabilitation and to enhance service delivery by providing an array of rehabilitation service options to society. The private-for-profit sector is a welcomed addition to this effort. Its presence must, however, be in the context of supplementing established services, not supplanting them—even a combined effort today would still fall short of reducing the current economic dependency of handicapped individuals.

A first step in the development of collaborative relationships should be the establishment of an agreement in principle between state agencies and an organization or consortium of private agencies. This agreement would include the factors: a reciprocal referral process, client placement, the development of facilities, and staff training.

Reciprocal Referral Process

In a reciprocal referral process (Griswold & Scott, 1979), the state agency would remain the principal agency to serve those who have no private support or as an alternative rehabilitation program when preferred by the consumer.

The province of the private agency is obviously with those individuals who can pay for such service, personally or through their insurance carrier or employer. The PFP agency also can provide services under contract to the SVR agency. The state agency can utilize private companies for psychological testing, vocational evaluation, counseling and guidance, on-the-job training, and placement. While each of these services is possible through the state agency, PFPs can augment these services. In cases where rehabilitation agencies find they are limited in manpower, it would be appropriate to hire this service from an external source.

Many states now find, as federal and state appropriations for rehabilitation have not kept pace with the cost of living, that there has been a gradual decrease in total counseling staff available for service. State legislatures traditionally support case service funds that go into direct client grants, as this is more politically palatable than the addition of state-supported counseling, guidance, and placement staff. This would in turn imply purchase of services external to the state program even though the end result would be higher overall expense to the public.

Private agencies can refer to the state clients who require services beyond those covered by workers' compensation laws or other insurance. A PFP company's responsibility may terminate, for example, with placement, while the client's rehabilitation needs could require periodic further intervention (counseling related to job retention, attendant care, dealing with psychological problems, etc.). A referral to the state agency would be appropriate at that time.

Mutual clients may also be those who have preexisting disabilities that have no relationship to the compensable injury and that may require additional rehabilitation services. If the private company is prohibited from service regarding the preexisting condition, a collaborative approach with the public agency may result in a more comprehensive solution. In addition, most state agencies have some specialized resources that can be made available to PFPs at lower cost than duplicating such resources in the private system. Georgia, for example, has established a state vocational assessment center that may be utilized by private agencies at cost.

Client Placement

One of the more critical rehabilitation services is client placement. Private agencies have taken a leadership role in establishing effective placement programs, particularly since their general philosophy is that a return to former employment is the strategy of choice (Welch, 1979). This has meant a history of service to business and industry that could be utilized by the public agency if a collaborative arrangement was established. Conversely, the public agency often has developed considerable placement contacts and may have established industrial accounts or productive relationships with the U.S. Employment Service. These openings can be made available in collaboration with private agencies for access by their clients seeking employment. As many private companies do not have a staff specialist and supportive equipment like word processing, videotape equipment, and occupational information systems such as state agencies have to facilitate the development of job-seeking skills and job-search behaviors, these might be made available to PFP agencies on a fee-for-use basis. Included in this referral package would be those clients referred to the state agency for Targeted Job Tax Credit eligibility. This federal provision allows companies to obtain tax credit for placement of individuals certified as vocationally handicapped by state rehabilitation agencies.

The Development of Facilities

A third area of common interest is rehabilitation facilities development. Traditionally, facilities have been developed through private charities and, in the last decade, through facility grant mechanisms by the state. While private agencies have not utilized facilities to a large degree, it would be appropriate for facilities to address some of the vocational evaluation and work adjustment needs of the private sector. In turn, the private sector could assist in securing private grants to develop the necessary service response by the rehabilitation facility.

In some larger industrial establishments it may be possible to establish vocational evaluation and work adjustment programs within an industrial plant if the volume of industrially disabled persons so warrants. Corporations that are committed to hiring individuals with disabilities may use that setting as a work entry point. Access to such a facility would be through both the private and public sectors.

Staff Training

Another area for collaboration would be the development of mutual training activities. Preservice training at the university level is usually in the areas of vocational evaluation, work adjustment, and rehabilitation counseling. There is, however, a strong need for mutual in-service training in which a consortium of private agencies and the public agency could share facilities, faculty, and training sessions. This would particularly enhance constructive relationships, the establishment of standards, and the beginning of an assurance of quality service to the community.

These are only some of the areas of potential cooperation. There are also current collaborative efforts between SVRs and PFPs in a number of states regarding counselor certification, participation in rehabilitation associations and conferences, and political action to assure appropriate funding for rehabilitation services.

Critical Issues

From the principle that a high degree of cooperation is desirable between the public and private rehabilitation sectors, some critical issues that must be faced in the next few years by all rehabilitation professionals can be derived. These include the following:

1. *Standards of ethics for rehabilitation professionals must be developed.* For too long there have been mutual accusations and recriminations between the public and private sectors suggesting that one is more ethically intact than the other. Some rehabilitation associations (for example, the Michigan Rehabilitation Association) have developed a standard of ethics for rehabilitation professionals. The National Association of Rehabilitation Professionals in the Private Sector (NARPPS) has also promulgated a standard (Scher, 1979). These efforts, fully embraced by both parties, can show the larger community that rehabilitation—both in the public and private sectors—does have professional standards and a code of ethics for the performance of duties.
2. *Public and private sectors must pool their resources to expand the scope of client services in the 1980s.* There currently are technological advances such as job engineering that should be implemented to develop requisite capacity within each state. There is a need to utilize all available current knowledge, techniques, and methods to realize the potential of disabled individuals. While it may not be possible for any one public or private agency to secure all such capacities, a statewide resource center accessible to both types of agencies would be beneficial. Just as public agencies may purchase services from the private sector, there often are sophisticated rehabilitation techniques available only through state agencies that could be purchased by private agencies.
3. *The nationwide effort by both public and private agencies to upgrade the staff qualifications for rehabilitation services should be encouraged.* The private sector has taken a leadership role in this effort primarily because they wish to make their services attractive and to demonstrate to the public the competency of their staff. State agencies, while wanting an equally attractive staff, have often been impeded by civil service regulations, cost containment activities, and in some cases union contracts from hiring and retaining the most qualified staff. SVR agencies have also suffered from prolonged internal debates over what staff is necessary for appro-

> priate services. The resolution of this problem seems to lie in having an array of different talents, but there is no national consensus in this direction. Legislation on certification for rehabilitation counselors has been introduced nationally and in some states. This may be a step in the right direction, but there still is a serious need to equate certification with competency. This effort can be advanced by cooperation between both sectors.

It is estimated that service is currently afforded only to a fraction of those who are vocationally handicapped and unable to find work without appropriate rehabilitation services. PFP and SVR agencies must work together to garner appropriate support for the funding of services to ensure that public and private costs for dependency are reduced and that the handicapped work force is able to reach its potential in employment and independence. This can only be done by collaboration between both groups based on a sensitive understanding of the positions of both parties and a willingness to reduce, if not eliminate, the vocational problems experienced by America's disabled population.

References

Bowe, F. *Rehabilitating America*. New York: Harper & Row, 1980.

Diamond, C. R., & Petkas, E. J. A state agency's view of private-for-profit rehabilitation. *Journal of Rehabilitation*, 1979, *45*(3), 30–31.

Griswold, P. P., & Scott, J. W. The state rehabilitation agency and private rehabilitation—A partnership long overdue. *Journal of Rehabilitation*, 1979, *45*(3), 32–33, 70.

Scher, P. L. NARPPS—Key to the survival of rehabilitation in the 1980s. *Journal of Rehabilitation*, 1979, *45*(13), 50–51, 74.

Welch, G. T. The relationship of rehabilitation with industry. *Journal of Rehabilitation*, 1979, *45*(3), 24–25.

3 Providing Rehabilitation Services to the Insurance Industry

Richard M. Keane

Introduction

This chapter will introduce the reader to the insurance industry as a consumer of rehabilitation services. Most rehabilitation professionals know very little about insurance prior to their employment in the private sector. Once privately employed, they find the maze of private bureaucracy as difficult to deal with as its counterpart in government agencies. All insurance companies are different. Each has different goals and objectives. Each has a different mix of business. Each company markets and services its products differently. No two companies are staffed alike. Despite all the differences, many private rehabilitation service providers approach all insurance companies using a similar sales presentation.

During the 1970s, benefit levels and costs related to workers' compensation increased at an unprecedented level. As companies struggled to contain costs, they turned to state/federal rehabilitation agencies and private nonprofit facilities. Neither was responsive. Private rehabilitation practitioners have been responsive. They have filled a critical need for the insurance industry. At the same time, the insurance industry has given life to private rehabilitation. They have paid millions of dollars for rehabilitation services. Overall, the insurance industry has paid the largest amount of money for private rehabilitation services (Eaton, 1979).

This chapter will explore the differences between different insurance companies and their needs. It will outline the differences between the types of insurance which might require rehabilitation services. It will describe what services are demanded and relate them to the structure of the insurance company. Just as a farm tractor company sells different sizes and types of equipment to Connecticut gentlemen farmers and huge Iowa farmers, so should private rehabilitation service providers adapt their services and marketing approaches for each prospective customer.

The Insurance Industry: An Overview

To understand the insurance industry's involvement in rehabilitation, it is necessary to understand the insurance industry. Few industries have impact on more lives, yet most Americans know very little about insurance company operations.

Insurance companies are financial institutions. They collect premiums, pay claims, and invest monies. For many companies, underwriting losses can coexist with net gains because of investments. For example, premiums for 1970 are collected and invested. When the last of the claims for that year are finally paid in 1985 and administrative costs are added, an underwriting loss (premium minus both claims and administrative costs) may have resulted. At the same time, investment income during those 15 years may have returned a net profit to the company. Whether it is a mutual company (returning a portion of profits to policyholders) or a stock company (returning a portion of profits to the stockholders), the insurance company must be conscious both of its policyholders as buyers of insurance and its investors as owners of the company and its assets.

Most people are not involved in insurance as an investment but rather as a protection against damages which occur as a result of events beyond their control. Automobile accidents, wind storms, medical problems, and death are just a few examples. Generally, the purchase of insurance is a subject of personal preference, but in some lines of insurance, it may be required by law. Workers' compensation, for example, is a required insurance for employers just as automobile insurance is required in a large number of states for owners of automobiles.

Insurance companies are organized in a number of ways but usually along product or function lines. A close look at any individual company makes it apparent that an organization is usually a combination of both product and function with an emphasis toward one. If the product line organization is predominant, similar types of insurance are grouped together with most of the company functions included within the product line groupings. For example, commercial lines insurance may include workers' compensation and commercial automobile. The underwriters, actuaries, and claims people will work in a single department serving the needs of those who buy commercial lines insurance. In the case of functional grouping, underwriters work in one department and claims people in another. Since many of the responsibilities link to other functional areas, it is very common to find strong liaison units or other means of cooperative working arrangements.

Regardless of corporate structure, all major companies will have a home office and separate field offices or their equivalent. The functions of the home-office staff and field-office staff are designed to provide the most effective claim services. If the company sells claim service as an important part of the insurance product, then the home office-field office relationship will be structured to provide full service in as many locations as possible. If pricing is the key factor in insurance sales, the company will probably control claims services from its home office or from a regional office. The claim departments or divisions need to work closely with the underwriting and sales staff to develop realistic and effective claim practices with insured people or companies. The home office functions will include almost all financial dealings, actuarial support, payroll, training centers, data processing, and senior management functions. Sales and claim support and second-level supervisory functions are also found in the home office or regional offices. The field offices are usually staffed by sales, engineering, personnel, and claim people. The field offices may have a manager of each function and that manager will often have a near complete authority with regard to the functions of his staff and equipment.

Insurer/Insured Relations: A Claim Department Concern

While a field office may become independent of home office assistance in the area of rehabilitation, it will never be independent of its responsibilities to policyholders and their employees.

Field-office staff in almost every insurance company answer to a number of authorities. The most important of these is the insured, the customer. In workers' compensation the insured may be a small "mom and pop" store or a huge multinational corporation doing business in the territory covered by the field office of that insurance company. Small companies may fear that their insurance premiums may be raised if additional outside services, such as rehabilitation, are purchased. Large corporations, on the other hand, by virtue of their contract with the insurance carrier, may be able to dictate how individual claims are handled. This may extend to the types of outside services purchased. Quite obviously, the purchaser of insurance feels strongly that the customer should have a say as to how its insurance company operates.

On occasion, a rehabilitation plan may even be abandoned because the insured company disapproves of it. In states where rehabilitation is not mandatory, this is always a possibility, especially with companies whose premiums are based on claim dollars paid over the life of the policy (and usually several years beyond). The employer (the insured) may disapprove of a rehabilitation plan for any number of reasons. Costs, precedents, and disagreement over the need are a few examples.

State agencies also dictate how workers' compensation claims will be handled. Industrial accident board staff, commissioners, and judges all evaluate an individual field office staff member's performance. On occasion, the insured may demand that a certain action take place in the file, while a workers' compensation commission may rule otherwise. This, of course, complicates the insurer/insured relationship which the claims person is expected to nurture.

Closing Files: Another Claim Department Concern

Home-office examiners and senior staff also influence the activities of the field-office staff. Company or claim department goals are used to measure a field office's performance. One example of a goal which is very important to insurance companies and very challenging to field offices is the back-log ratio. This ratio is the relationship between the number of new lost-time accidents which remain open in the office at the end of the month. For example, an office may have 1,000 files open at the beginning of the month. It opens 100 new files during the month and closes 100. At the end of the month, 1,000 files still remain open. This provides a ten to one back-log ratio. The reason that back-log ratios are so important is that the longer a file is open and has issues unresolved, the more expensive it becomes. Long-term disabilities often result in psychological problems when an injured worker is left to worry about his or her future. These problems may become more serious than the original injury itself.

The importance of closing files should be understood by rehabilitation counselors who seek to begin rehabilitation services early. As is widely known, beginning early avoids complications as a disabled person goes through the stages of dealing with disability. The same complications that present rehabilitation obstacles can increase claim and medical costs for the insurance company. The sooner an injured worker is provided with rehabilitation services designed to return him to work, the sooner the other legal and medical issues can be resolved and the file closed.

The reason many adjusters or supervisors wait so long to refer a case is their belief that all disability issues will resolve spontaneously. Rehabilitation services take months to provide. If a case is resolved quickly without rehabilitation services, then the case can be closed quickly. Every year just enough of the very tough cases which might have been long-term problems resolve themselves seemingly miraculously. These infrequent "miracles" are enough to keep the spark of hope alive and to keep potential rehabilitation referrals in file cabinets in the claims office.

Insurance companies spend millions of dollars on rehabilitation services, yet many argue that not enough is being done (Deneen & Hessellund, 1981). In the few states where rehabilitation is mandated by law for injured workers unable to return to their usual and customary work after medical recovery, there is no alternative. Cost effective, timely rehabilitation services are provided to bring about the earliest possible closing date for a file. Since the money being spent is usually the insured's money, the insurance company really has two mandates: the insured demands that the earliest possible closure of the file be an objective, while the state demands a rehabilitation program which will result in the injured workers' return to work.

In those states where rehabilitation is not mandatory, a different set of pressures exist. The insured still wants the file closed as soon as possible, but pressure may be placed by the claimant and/or his doctor or attorney to delay the return to work as long as possible. The injured worker fears the loss of benefits and often believes that he or she would be unable to get benefits reinstated if the return to work is not a permanent solution to the problem. Doctors fear medical malpractice suits. They are also given very inaccurate information about an injured worker's job, which means that they honestly believe an injured worker cannot return to work at a later date when, in fact, he or she may be able to do so.

As many rehabilitation service providers know, it is usually necessary to get a clear indication of what a disabled person's restrictions are. The attending physician should be an excellent source of information concerning these restrictions. Unfortunately, the attending physician may or may not be able to clearly state an injured worker's restrictions functionally until someone provides the job description of the person's former job or of any job to which the injured worker may be able to return using transferable skills.

Insurance Products

In addition to understanding the organizational structure of insurance companies and their claim departments' concerns, it is important to understand some basic elements about the insurance products which generate the claims. Each state and each company dictate what is covered (Wales & Ideson, 1977). Optional coverage is also possible on some types of insurance policies.

Workers' Compensation

Workers' compensation insurance is the result of a compromise between an employee's right to sue for damages resulting from a personal injury at work and an employer's right to use defenses of contributory negligence and acceptance of risk (Larson, 1979). Prior to workers' compensation legislation which began in the United States in 1911, injured workers found themselves at a distinct disadvantage in trying to sue and collect for damages while, at the same time, trying to preserve their jobs (Wales & Ideson, 1977). Today the vast majority of workers in the United States are covered under state workers' compensation legislation. In addition to each state having a workers' compensation law, separate programs on the federal level cover millions of additional workers. An example is the Longshoremen and Harbor Workers' Act (often referred to as the USL Act) which covers these workers regardless of their state of domicile and where the injury occurs.

There are similarities in the benefits provided under all workers' compensation laws. Before considering these, however, the reader should carefully note that all state workers' compensation acts are different (Chamber of Commerce, 1982). Unfortunately, many rehabilitation professionals in the private and public sectors have viewed all clients covered under workers' compensation policies as having identical benefits. Actually, two injured workers covered under the same workers' compensation act could be receiving very different benefits just as two injured workers from different states will almost certainly have different benefits. It is not uncommon for an injured worker covered under the workers' compensation act of one state to move to another state. A rehabilitation counselor called upon to provide rehabilitation services under these circumstances must consider the benefits to which this injured worker is entitled (Eaton, 1979). Almost without exception, the benefits are those of the jurisdiction under which the injury was originally covered.

There are three general types of payments that can be made on a workers' compensation file: claim, medical, and expense. The following pages will explain the differences. The failure to understand these categories has caused many problems between rehabilitation professionals and insurance claims people.

Claim Benefits. Claims benefits include a number of different benefits which sometimes seem blended together. The temporary total (TT) disability payment is the most common. It is paid to a worker who is temporarily totally unable to work due to the injury. In a number of states, this benefit is paid indefinitely, while in other states it is paid until the injured worker reaches a level referred to as Maximum Medical Improvement (MMI) or Permanent and Stationary (P and S). At this point a worker who is unable to return to work would receive either "permanent partial" or "permanent total" disability payments.

The permanent partial (PP) disability payment is the second most common type of claim benefit. Workers who suffer an injury which results in a permanent loss of function will usually be compensated, at least in part, for their loss. How the payments are determined differ substantially from state to state. In some states a chart is used to determine the values of any specific disabilities. In other states, a medical report determines the loss of function as it relates to the body as a whole. For example, a 20% loss of use of the dominant hand might equate to a 5% loss of the body as a whole. This is then translated into a dollar amount to be paid to the claimant. How the payments are made also differs markedly. In some states, the payment is made periodically for a predetermined length of time. Another type of permanent partial payment system is being used in Florida. This "wage loss" system measures permanent loss as lost wages following an injured worker's completion of rehabilitation and return to work. For each week that an injured worker receives less than the former wages, the insurance company or self-insured employer pays two-thirds of the difference up to a legal maximum for a period of up to 525 weeks.

Temporary partial (TP) disability payments are made to an injured worker who is able to work part time or full time but at a lower rate of pay. For each week of earnings below the average earned prior to the injury, the injured worker is entitled to two-thirds of the difference up to a legal maximum (usually the temporary total rate) until the worker is able to return to his usual rate of pay. This benefit is an excellent one to use in a rehabilitation program. It allows the worker to try a new job, possibly at an entry-level position, with a minimal loss of income. Unfortunately, many rehabilitation counselors are not aware of this benefit, and it is not available in every state.

Permanent total disability (PTD) payments are generally made to an injured worker whose disability is so disabling that it prevents a return to gainful employment. Rehabilitation counselors familiar with state/federal vocational rehabilitation system caseloads find that this classification is used far too often in workers' compensation cases. Many disabled workers are classified as PTD because of the combination of the physical disability and the pain symptomology. Pain behaviors are often the key factors in a doctor's decision to rate an injured worker as unable to do any gainful work. Some states declare people permanently and totally disabled if they suffer certain injury types. Connecticut, for example, declares a person permanently and totally disabled if the injured worker loses the use of both legs or both arms or both eyes. Even though such injured workers may return to work earning as much or more as before the injury, they are entitled to permanent total disability payments for life.

Vocational rehabilitation services are another claim benefit. A tremendous amount of flexibility is built into vocational rehabilitation benefits in most states. In the few states which mandate vocational rehabilitation services for injured workers who are unable to return to their usual and customary work, the degree of flexibility is lessened. In the 40 plus other states, however, different companies will provide very different vocational rehabilitation services. The company's claim handling philosophy, their marketing strategy, and their staffing pattern all dictate how they approach vocational rehabilitation services.

Generally, vocational rehabilitation benefits include payment of outside rehabilitation service providers' bills, evaluation costs, training costs, and the costs of tools and equipment for a new profession. In some cases, insurance companies pay to modify a job site to help an injured worker return to work. In other cases, an insurance company might pay the cost of setting up an injured worker in self-employment.

Medical Benefits. Medical benefits cover hospitalization, doctors' bills, medical rehabilitation, wheelchairs, orthoses, prostheses, and a variety of other items. Medical benefits cover a visiting physical or occupational therapist when it is recommended by the doctor and approved by the insurance company. This is sometimes preferable to paying high mileage charges for an injured worker who is traveling a considerable distance to get the same service. Whirlpool baths, special beds, adaptive appliances, and innovative transportation solutions can all be made available under medical benefits.

A rehabilitation counselor working on a workers' compensation case should be certain of what is covered as a medical benefit because there are major differences from one jurisdiction to another. For example, in one jurisdiction a paraplegic may be entitled to automobile hand controls and a wheelchair. In another jurisdiction, a similar injury might entitle the injured worker to modification of his or her home and assistance in buying a specially prepared van. In addition, two insurance companies may offer vastly different services under medical benefits, both meeting the dictates of the same state law. As an example, Company A may pay for a ramp on a paraplegic's home and hand controls for his or her car. Company B may build an addition to the home with an adapted bathroom, wider doorways, and ramps. They also may advance the injured worker the money to purchase a more dependable car, in addition to paying for hand controls.

Medical rehabilitation involves a vast array of services and equipment which are related to restoration of the physical and psychological well-being of the injured worker. Travel expenses, prosthetic appliances, wheelchairs, hospital beds, and whirlpool baths are all examples. Rehabilitation counselors working in the private sector should not hesitate to inquire of claims personnel exactly what is covered. Also, if a rehabilitation counselor honestly believes a specific service or piece of equipment would substantially help an injured worker to return to work, a claim supervisor/adjuster may make exceptions to general rules.

Expense Payments. There are a number of payments which are made under this category. If an independent medical examination is required to determine the extent of an injured worker's disability, this is paid as an expense. Special claim investigation expenses, legal expenses, and certain expenses for testimony in workers' compensation cases may also be paid as expenses.

These administrative expenses should not be confused with expenses that are related to the provision of rehabilitation services. If a private rehabilitation counselor bills an insurance company for its travel, housing, or office expenses, these will be paid as a claim item. They are not called expense items in the workers' compensation file.

Legislation for Cost Control

In the late 1970s, the sharply rising costs of workers' compensation for both employers and insurers generated huge increases in premiums. Even with premiums raised by 100% and more, workers' compensation insurance became very unprofitable. An examination of the reasons uncovered a number of causes, which included sharply rising weekly benefit rates, liberalization of workers' compensation coverage, and rising medical costs (Hatch, 1979).

Some states changed legislation to combat the problems. Florida is a good example. Because of its runaway workers' compensation premium increases, a major revamping of Florida's workers' compensation law was accomplished and took effect August 1, 1979. This resulted in two successive decreases in workers' compensation premiums. Essentially, the new legislation sought to put a larger percentage of the claim dollars in the hands of the more severely injured worker and to provide a strong incentive to the less severely disabled to return to work. Florida's changes included the mandating of vocational rehabilitation services for injured workers who are unable to return to their usual jobs. Previously, many injured workers sought lump sum settlements for their injuries. This system provided a disincentive for workers to return to work. The present system provides strong incentive to both the injured worker and the insurance company to begin rehabilitation efforts early (Waters, 1981).

In many states where rehabilitation is not mandated by law, rehabilitation is being employed to reduce the amount of money which would be owed if the injured worker did not return to work. However, some state laws contain sections which tend to reduce the cost effectiveness of rehabilitation. For example, in Kansas, a court ruled that a successful rehabilitation program would not change an injured worker's settlement to partial benefits if he or she remained unable to do the job held prior to the injury (Antwi, 1980). A college student working summers in a factory might receive an injury which precludes continuing in that job. The student returns to school, graduates, and goes on to a career in a profession. The new professional remains entitled to benefits in the state of Kansas if he or she is unable to do the work engaged in during the summer employment, according to this decision.

Workers' compensation rehabilitation, then, is greatly affected by both legislative developments and court decisions at the state level.

No-Fault Automobile Insurance

While workers' compensation cases make up the bulk of private rehabilitation counselors' case loads, other types of insurance claims are referred for services. No-fault automobile insurance, which provides benefits for injured policyholders, has provided a large number of cases for rehabilitation professionals in a number of states. Generally, only those states with the high mandatory Personal Injury Protection (PIP) coverage will provide substantial numbers of files. Historically, Michigan, New York, New Jersey, and Pennsylvania have led the nation in providing rehabilitation services for injured automobile accident victims. Most states allow policyholders to purchase higher limits of insurance which means files may be referred in any state with no-fault automobile insurance programs.

It is worth noting that no-fault cases may involve injured people with no competitive work history. In workers' compensation cases this is highly unlikely. (The only exceptions in workers' compensation might involve sheltered workshop employees in jurisdictions which do not consider these employees as students.) Automobile accidents cause brain damage and/or spinal cord injuries at a higher rate than workers' compensation cases. These cases tend to be more costly and involve more lengthy rehabilitation plans than do workers' compensation cases.

Long-Term Disability (LTD) Insurance

Long-term disability (LTD) cases are being referred for rehabilitation services with increasing frequency. LTD benefits may be part of an individual disability insurance package or part of a group benefit available through an employer or a professional affiliation. LTD policies are the product of a very competitive and ever-more-highly regulated line of insurance. To sell policies, insurance companies may offer very liberal benefits. For example, benefits may initially be paid to a worker who cannot return to his or her specific job, despite the worker's ability to do a wide variety of jobs paying higher wages. Generally, after a certain amount of time, the insurance policy continues to provide benefits only if a worker is unable to do any type of work.

The required wording of policies often frustrates the use of rehabilitation to help injured workers return to jobs. LTD benefit recipients may not be required to cooperate with rehabilitation programs. Even more frustrating, they may need not accept a job upon completion of the rehabilitation program. This problem is partly caused by late referrals for rehabilitation services. Most LTD policies provide benefits once the injured person has been disabled more than six months. For this reason, most insurance companies will refer LTD files well after six months of disability.

Despite the frustrations, LTD cases are being sought by many private rehabilitation service providers because as competition grows in private rehabilitation, new sources of referrals are required. LTD cases, once considered a poor substitute for workers' compensation cases, are now treasured by many rehabilitation professionals.

Liability Insurance

Liability cases can be generated under a number of different insurance policies. A general liability policy may be purchased by the owner of a business. A homeowner's policy will usually provide limited liability coverage for the homeowner. A manufacturer may purchase product liability insurance. Automobile policies provide liability coverage even under no-fault policies.

Liability cases are still a small minority of referrals for rehabilitation services. This has been true because of the adversarial relationship which exists between the injured person (and his or her attorney) and the insurance company. For example, a customer is hit by a can of paint falling from a high shelf. This customer suffers brain damage which necessitates lengthy rehabilitation. The injured person and his attorney will try to present the injuries as permanent impediments to any sort of normal life. Proof of this before a jury would make the case a very valuable one.

Rehabilitation services tend to mitigate the damages, thereby reducing the value of the case. The consequence has been a general reluctance on the part of insurance companies to use rehabilitation for injured people who have brought liability claims against them. They claim that attorneys will be unresponsive to the attempts at rehabilitation. Fortunately, this thinking is beginning to be disproven by successful rehabilitation attempts in liability cases.

In the past, most liability cases were settled by the payment of a lump-sum settlement. Attorneys received a percentage, and the remainder was given to the person who suffered the loss. Very frequently, the recipient of such a lump-sum settlement would use the money quickly and inappropriately. During the past decade a new means of paying settlements has become prominent. Insurance companies are paying for annuities which pay the injured person over his or her lifetime. Attorneys receive their fees, but injured people are able to receive much more money over a longer period of time. These structured settlements may pay a fixed amount at the beginning and periodic payments thereafter.

Rehabilitation services are sometimes required in these settlements. Insurance companies may offer or be required by the court to provide services which restore a person to as high a level of functioning as possible. In other instances, rehabilitation services may be used by insurance companies or self-insured defendants to demonstrate a willingness to help an injured person. A rehabilitation provider may be called upon to offer such services.

Claim Department Organization

Learning about insurance companies, their products, and their structure is a start. Learning more about insurance people is the next and most important step in providing rehabilitation services for insurance companies. A number of surveys done in the past few years have shown that, generally, people employed in the insurance industry are not trusted. Most claims people are not the mechanical, unfeeling bureaucrats envisioned by the average person, however. In fact, claims people are often very similar in background to professionals in many fields in manufacturing, government, and social services. The backgrounds of claims people may include law, medicine, social work, teaching, sports, and even rehabilitation counseling.

Claim departments tend to pay salaries in the middle range for all jobs requiring similar experiences. A person who handles claims probably feels underpaid and overworked just as millions of other American workers do (U.S. Department of Labor, 1978).

Most annual salaried claims people hold college degrees (U.S. Department of Labor, 1977). Their preparation may vary widely, but generally they have demonstrated an ability to integrate facts, weigh alternative solutions, and make decisions. As in any other field, some are very capable and dedicated, while others appear overwhelmed and unmotivated by their jobs.

Some insurance companies put claims people through extensive and ongoing training programs. Other companies avoid the costs of training by primarily or only hiring experienced claims people. In either type of company, the quality of work is a function of many variables including the individual's interest in the work and his or her self-esteem.

Some companies prefer to make their claims people experts in a particular line of insurance. Such a person may handle only workers' compensation claims, for example. Other companies have assigned a number of different types of insurance claims to their staff to give them broad backgrounds. These people may handle workers' compensation, automobile damage, general liability, and group insurance, for example. There is merit to each approach, but it is important to understand that there are differences in the preparation of claims people. Learning about these differences may be the counselor's key to working successfully with an insurance company.

One experience is shared by many claims people all across the United States. They have been inundated by the flood of private rehabilitation service providers. The growth of the private rehabilitation industry and the necessity to market the services personally have created a problem. Very qualified rehabilitation service providers are unable to attract referrals because they are unable to present their materials to the right people. To be successful, private rehabilitation agency people must be sensitive to the heavy workloads of claims people. They must also recognize that they may be the most recent in a long line of people selling similar services. Persistence pays off for those who are patient and sensitive. Persistence, however, may forever doom to failure the insensitive seekers of referrals. Those who receive referrals will usually be those who quietly present their materials and loudly demonstrate their results!

In-House Rehabilitation Programs

One of the early responses to the large increase in workers' compensation was the change in insurance company cost control programs. Liberty Mutual Insurance Company staffed many of its offices with rehabilitation nurses who worked to reduce both medical costs and the amount of time lost from work. This became an important aspect of the claim handling procedures of this company (Lewin, Ramseur, & Sink, 1979).

In 1972, Insurance of North American (INA) spun off International Rehabilitation Associates (IRA), the largest private-for-profit rehabilitation provider during the 1970s and early 1980s. They provided services not only for their parent company but for other insurance and self-insurers as well. This daring move at such an early stage in the development of workers' compensation rehabilitation points out the company's accurate perception of the depth and breadth of changes that the insurance industry faced in the 1970s and faces in the 1980s. Today, over 60 IRA offices, staffed primarily with medically trained personnel who receive additional training in vocational rehabilitation, provide a full range of rehabilitation services not only to INA but to hundreds of other insurance companies and self-insured companies.

As the cost control measures of the 1970s gained credibility, they became necessary to compete in the workers' compensation market. Dozens of large and small insurance companies added medically trained staff as either medical representatives or rehabilitation nurses. Home office staff positions were established, and special programs were added in medical and vocational rehabilitation. Training in rehabilitation for field and home office employees is conducted by in-house and outside rehabilitation specialists.

There are a number of possible advantages in having an in-house rehabilitation program. Four are listed here. First, by having such a program, an insurance company can demand and get timely services. Second, insurance companies can control who works on cases, thereby getting exactly the services demanded. Third, it is cost effective to have in-house rehabilitation staff working on a minimum number of cases. Fourth, in some jurisdictions, the law requires rehabilitation services to be provided in such a manner that it is most effective to do this with staff familiar with the philosophy and needs of the insurance company.

It is important to note that there are also disadvantages to having in-house staff working on rehabilitation plans. In some states, it is highly probable that attorneys or others may object to an insurance staff member working on a rehabilitation plan. It is also probable that injured workers may find it difficult to work with a representative of the same company, who they may find threatening in a legal environment. A company also loses the flexibility of being able to refer cases to specialists who deal with one type of case better than another.

Like claim departments themselves, rehabilitation programs come in a wide variety of types. The different purposes for the programs dictate different staffing patterns. Those companies that are most interested in the medical aspects of rehabilitation try to staff their programs with medically oriented people. Those companies that are interested in vocational rehabilitation as the focal point of the program will hire staff who have had training and/or experience in that area.

The type and extent of the program set up by any specific insurance company has usually depended upon either the size of the company or the state mandates with which they must work. Two of the largest writers of workers' compensation insurance each have over 100 rehabilitation nurses/medical representatives nationwide. These staff members are located in jurisdictions mandating rehabilitation services, as well as in jurisdictions which tend to discourage vocational rehabilitation services. Smaller insurance companies may do a large percentage of their business in one or two states. The laws of the states they work in may dictate the composition of their field staff. In one state they may have rehabilitation nurses and/or rehabilitation counselors, while in another state, this same company may have claim technicians only. Small insurance companies which provide workers' compensation coverage primarily for local companies usually do not have to deal with large national insureds who expect similar service in every state in which they do business.

Many differences become apparent when comparing the medical and vocational rehabilitation programs of individual insurance companies. Most companies have long since learned that a small percentage of their total number of lost-time accidents represent a large percentage of their claim dollars. A variety of methods have been employed to address this fact. The in-house rehabilitation program is one of these.

Insurance Rehabilitation Referrals

Understanding the insurance company's structure is extremely important for those selling rehabilitation services. Many believe incorrectly that all home offices of insurance companies dictate which private rehabilitation providers will be used and when. This is very often not true, as with The Travelers Insurance Company. A rehabilitation agency anxious to sell their services to insurance companies should learn how the insurance companies are organized to provide claim services. Basically, there are four options.

First, the company may control which rehabilitation agencies will be used and on which cases they will be used. The home office in this case will probably carry a duplicate file and even supervise directly some activities on the more serious cases. The field office will meet with the claimant and carry out the dictates of the home office.

Second, the home office may approve or disapprove of the available rehabilitation agencies but allow the field offices to choose the cases on which the services will be used.

Third, the home office may dictate what cases require vocational rehabilitation service but allow the field office to select the provider of rehabilitation services.

The fourth possibility is probably the most common. The home office allows the field office to select both the rehabilitation provider and the cases on which the services will be used. Obviously, in this system the home-office function is to train field-office staff to use effectively available rehabilitation services. Most companies in this category spend a significant amount of time training their staff to understand what rehabilitation services can be expected from a private rehabilitation provider.

Many companies do not fit neatly into any of these four categories. In one part of the country, the company may follow rehabilitation cases carefully from the home office. For another part of the country, its field office may be entirely responsible for the rehabilitation of injured workers. Ultimately, the best source of information about the company's policy is the person who refers the file for services.

The Largest Workers' Compensation Insurance Companies

There are several hundred insurance companies that provide workers' compensation insurance. The largest five of these received close to one-third of all the premiums collected by insurance companies in the United States for workers' compensation insurance in 1979 (Best, 1981). All of the insurance companies providing workers' compensation must service their customers in some way. Each company has a program very different from the others and updates it regularly to meet the demands of the law and the marketplace.

The next few pages will describe the specific direction of each of the largest five companies as they operate in the early 1980s. Much of the material in these pages represents the philosophy of insurance companies.

The reader should be aware of the differences that may exist between a company's policy and the actual practice of any of its field offices.

The five companies discussed here provide insurance coverage in almost every jurisdiction other than the monopolistic states.[1] There are companies that provide insurance in one or several states only. The way in which these companies are structured may be different than the structure of the larger company doing business in the same state.

Liberty Mutual

Liberty Mutual Insurance Company, the nation's largest writer of workers' compensation insurance, has centralized responsibility and monitors its most expensive files in the home office (Best, 1981). It works quickly on potentially expensive files to help resolve problems. Rehabilitation nurses in the field coordinate medical services and help injured workers in their recovery. The rapport developed between the rehabilitation nurses and the injured workers often helps the workers get through difficult periods in their recovery.

Liberty Mutual hires rehabilitation nurses full and part time. These staff members are registered nurses who provide medical management and cost-control services. They spend much time learning about community services, and they use them for their claimants. This company's rehabilitation nurses primarily focus on the medical aspects of their cases. They have developed considerable expertise in coordinating vocational rehabilitation services provided by outside service providers. Since they represent policyholders who pay over 8% of national workers' compensation premiums, it is important to understand clearly how they expect rehabilitation services to be provided. Liberty Mutual has chosen not to hire and train vocational rehabilitation service providers in almost all of their locations. Although they do have many staff knowledgeable in the area of vocational rehabilitation, they are buying rehabilitation services outside the company. Not only their size but their expertise makes them an excellent customer because of the preparatory work by their nursing staff. Their staff has a strong foundation in medical and vocational rehabilitation principles.

A unique program of the Liberty Mutual Insurance Company in the area of insurance rehabilitation has been its rehabilitation clinic. For a number of years, the company has transported severely disabled workers to the clinic from all over the United States. Even today, although not as cost effective, it provides the company with an opportunity to continue work in rehabilitation engineering. Very clearly, the home office is extremely

[1]State fund insurance companies are not included in this discussion. California, Colorado, Arizona, New York, and other states have state funds which compete with insurance companies. Wyoming, West Virginia, Washington, North Dakota, Nevada, and Ohio are states in which the state fund is the only insurance company providing workers' compensation. These six states are known as monopolistic states with regard to workers' compensation insurance.

important in this company's centralized handling of serious injury cases.

Despite the number of rehabilitation nurses employed by Liberty Mutual, it has for many years maintained a home-office staff to examine a large number of field files on a regular basis. Their home-office supervision of workers' compensation files is much closer than is normal for many of their competitors. There is considerable direct communication between the home office and field-office staff on specific issues on many files. It is not uncommon for a home-office staff person to fly to a location anywhere in the United States to help provide services to the disabled claimant.

During the 1970s, the names of Liberty Mutual's rehabilitation staff members were often found on the programs of conferences held throughout the United States on the subject of rehabilitation and the injured worker. The head of their program, George Sawyer, became known as an authority on insurance rehabilitation during the 1970s. The intimate involvement in files by their home-office staff, and the experience gained with their rehabilitation nurse program, provided them with unique insights into the dynamics of these disability cases (Sawyer, 1978).

Aetna Life and Casualty Insurance Company

Aetna Life and Casualty, the second largest writer of workers' compensation insurance with about 6% of the national premium, has a different type of rehabilitation program (Best, 1981). They began adding rehabilitation nurses in the late 1970s and early 1980s. Their handling of workers' compensation cases has involved considerable use of outside rehabilitation agencies for both medical management and vocational rehabilitation. Their home-office staff has done a good job of locating, evaluating, and using the best of the rehabilitation services available in the community.

In the 1980s their program will employ more rehabilitation nurses, which will mean fewer referrals for medical management and better referrals for vocational rehabilitation services. Their size and aggressive posture in the market makes them a coveted customer for the rehabilitation service provider.

The Travelers Insurance Company

The rehabilitation programs of The Travelers Insurance Company, the third largest writer of workers' compensation, involve the largest number of full-time medical representative/rehabilitation nurses employed by an insurance company.[2] In the late 1970s, the company began hiring job-placement spe-

[2]Editors' note. The author, employed by The Travelers Insurance Company, has appropriately dealt at more length with this company's in-house rehabilitation programs, based on his personal familiarity with them.

cialists and rehabilitation counselors. In 1981, 20 rehabilitation-counselor-trained staff were working in Florida and other active rehabilitation states. The company feels that these people are necessary additions to its workers' compensation staff in the effort to meet the mandates of state laws.

The Travelers has been very active in vocational rehabilitation, in addition to its work in medical rehabilitation. A number of innovative programs have helped them to increase the percentage of injured workers who return to work. One of the most widely used innovations is the Job Readiness Workshop. This is basically an adaption of job-seeking skills training to meet the unique needs of injured workers. The program has used both the compassion of workers' compensation staff and the flexibility of the insurance industry to meet the needs of people covered by this type of insurance.

Job Readiness Workshops combine the teaching of resume writing, application completion, and interviewing skills with the benefits of small group meetings to solve problems. Injured workers suffer from all the fears and anxieties of disabled people, but they are also subject to a set of problems uniquely associated with workers' compensation. Their fear of doing or saying "the wrong thing" and their misunderstandings concerning their rights under the law are just two areas discussed by the participants within the workshop context. The workshop provides an opportunity to express what they may have feared even thinking about prior to the workshop. This aspect of the workshop has contributed greatly to improve communication between the insurance company and the injured worker.

One of the key functions of the workshop is to help injured workers help themselves. As injured workers are shown methods of finding and soliciting jobs, they also gain confidence in their ability to compete in the job market for which they had previously felt unprepared. Many of the participants in these workshops report improved self-confidence. As rehabilitation counselors know, this is a vital necessity for any man or woman who has suffered the physical and emotional trauma associated with disability.

The workshops have returned about 30 percent of their participants to jobs directly. Approximately 15 percent have been helped to identify job goals which require further training or assistance. Others have been successfully weaned from extensive medical care. Since the participants are selected for the workshop because they have not been successful in their efforts to return to work or overcome serious problems, the 45-percent success rate is quite significant.

There are two special features of the Job Readiness Workshops. First, the overall coordination of the workshop is the responsibility of an insurance company staff person while the workshop itself is conducted by a rehabilitation consultant who is hired for this purpose. This consultant may come from either the private or public rehabilitation sector. The consultant's role is to conduct the exercises, to teach job-seeking skills, and to provide liaison with those providing follow-up services. The consultants work either for a fee per workshop or for a fee per claimant. The details of responsibilities are worked out for each workshop and are dependent upon the skills of the rehabilitation provider and the demands of the law covering the injured workers in the particular location.

The second special feature of these workshops is The Travelers Insurance Company's desire to get other insurance companies involved in them. In one Florida workshop, injured workers from several different insurance companies were grouped together. The workshop demonstrated that this is a viable arrangement. This approach makes the workshop available in areas of the country where no one company could conduct a workshop by itself for as many as eight to 12 workers. By prorating the expenses, several small companies can afford to run workshops on a regular basis. This also allows companies with lesser degrees of expertise in rehabilitation to benefit from companies with more extensive expertise.

The Travelers has been sharing its training materials with other insurance companies in an effort to have others consider conducting their own workshop. The training materials consist of a videocassette tape and a manual. They have been displayed at intercompany meetings and have been made available to companies individually. The hope is that the sharing of such programs will further enhance the development of rehabilitation services by insurance companies.

Very few companies have demonstrated an interest in sharing the responsibilities of a workshop or independently producing them thus far. Basically, there are two reasons why other companies have not adopted this program. The first involves the cycles of the insurance industry. These cycles, although financial in nature, affect many aspects of insurance company operations. As interest rates climb, competition for premium dollars increases. Increased competition causes lower prices, bigger advertising budgets, and an emphasis on making distinctions between companies and their products. Each company wants to sell as much of its product as possible. It is highly improbable that one company will adopt the program of another during this highly competitive portion of the cycle. Those who do will give the program a new look so that it is not associated with the originator of the idea. The second reason the workshops have not been adopted quickly is the belief by most insurance companies that the concept is too expensive and time-consuming for claims operations. Few claims people truly understand the anguish and suffering of a disabled worker who is struggling to return to his or her normal life. For some of these disabled people extraordinary measures are often necessary.

Insurance Company of North America (INA)

INA, the fourth largest writer of workers' compensation insurance in the United States is technically a general corporation rather than an insurance company (Best, 1981). This general corporation owns a number of companies which perform insurance and rehabilitation functions, among others. INA was the leader in developing the private rehabilitation field with its introduction of International Rehabilitation Associates (IRA). IRA leads the private rehabilitation field in a number of categories. It is the largest rehabilitation company; it has consistently advertised more heavily on a national basis than its competitors; and it has brought the most automated, computer-assisted program into the early 1980s. Its computer programs do billing, provide customers with details about their files, and do quick assessments to rate success probability for the individual injured worker. Originally lead by George Welch, a charismatic leader in rehabilitation, IRA is now shifting away from its dependence on charisma to a more business-like stance. For example, they have developed new cost containment products and tools to open up new products.

IRA has also been a leader in following legislative changes and in speaking out for and against legislation affecting the provision of rehabilitation services. IRA's marketing and support services have been models for other private rehabilitation providers. IRA has demonstrated versatility and persistence in seeking rehabilitation referrals in long-term disability and no-fault insurance. INA uses IRA almost exclusively for rehabilitation services, although INA does have some nurses who monitor medical costs as part of its cost control program.

Hartford Insurance Group

The fifth largest workers' compensation insurer is the Hartford Insurance Group, a conservative insurance company, but certainly not a backward one. It has a staff of rehabilitation nurses located in strategically located offices. As the need arises, the claims offices use rehabilitation service providers as much, if not more, than three of the four largest writers of workers' compensation insurance. This is an effective company in the area of rehabilitation. They believe in using the best available services to return disabled workers to jobs and to reduce their liability in workers' compensation claims. An advertisement in the *Wall Street Journal* (December 6, 1982) featuring the Hartford's Rehabilitation Program probably indicates their eagerness to continue improvements in their rehabilitation services.

Rehabilitation Company Subsidiaries

A number of insurance companies are developing subsidiaries which are selling rehabilitation services. Among the 20 largest writers of workers' compensation premiums, no less than four are operating rehabilitation subsidiaries. INA operates IRA, Continental Insurance Company operates Underwriters Adjusting Company (UAC), Kemper Insurance Group operates National Loss Control Service Corporation (NATLSCO), and The Travelers Insurance Company operates Constitution Rehabilitation Company (CRC). IRA has developed internationally, covering its area in the United States quite well. The other three are developing their service areas as the demand grows. It is also interesting to note that, except for INA, each of the parent corporations, either directly or indirectly, continues to use outside rehabilitation services extensively to return injured workers to jobs. This results from parent company decisions not to expand the subsidiaries too quickly into areas where the demand has not been demonstrated. Each of the companies varies the number of files referred to outside services as dictated by its staffing pattern for that area.

It is highly doubtful that any major insurer will attempt to completely end its need for outside rehabilitation services in the immediate future. It is not cost-effective to hire rehabilitation staff to work on every possible case. It is far more effective to have the staff member handle a manageable number of cases and then supplement staff work with services provided by outside rehabilitation agencies (Sawyer, 1981). Obviously, as the subsidiary of each parent company grows, there is the possibility that a larger percentage of the cases referred by these companies will be referred to the subsidiary.

Countering this tendency, most companies will grow at a pace consistent with the increasing demand for outside services. In some states, it may not be profitable to operate a private rehabilitation company as a subsidiary with the large overhead costs associated with national operations.

Self-Insured Companies

Those interested in providing services in the private-for-profit market should also be aware of another trend. Many large corporations are choosing self-insurance rather than purchasing an insurance policy. Small companies are able to become self-insured by joining associations of smaller companies and pooling their resources.

The growth of the self-insurance market generally means more outside services are necessary. The difficulty has been, however, that many risk managers (those responsible for processing insurance claims) have been unaware of the need for rehabilitation services. It is necessary, therefore, to sell services to such companies by first convincing them of the need for rehabilitation services in workers' compensation cases. Free training helps in this effort. Once this is done, then rehabilitation services may actually be sold on specific cases.

The self-insured market is growing rapidly, and the need for outside services is growing with it. Although it is considerably more time-consuming to make service calls to a large number of self-insured companies than to one insurance company, those who spend the extra time may develop a steady source of referrals.

Marketing Services to Insurance Companies

Assuming that all of the top 20 workers' compensation insurers are presently buying at least some rehabilitation services outside their corporation, and assuming that rehabilitation is cost effective in insurance cases, then it can be concluded that there is considerable work for many private rehabilitation service providers. The task for those interested in this field is to identify correctly the needs of the various insurance companies and to tailor services to meet the needs of these companies.

In the mid and late 1970s, hundreds of rehabilitation counselors moved into the private for-profit rehabilitation field. Many assumed that sheer determination and hard work would bring success. This simplistic view of this burgeoning business of private rehabilitation resulted in a number of companies going out of business before they had an opportunity to test the market.

In reality, successful private rehabilitation enterprise requires skill in both marketing and the provision of rehabilitation services. A private rehabilitation agency which cannot attract and hold new business cannot provide quality services. Conversely, an agency which can bring in referrals with its marketing staff but cannot satisfy the referring company with adequate services will eventually lose its sources of referrals. Then how is the ideal company staffed to meet both marketing and service needs?

The larger private rehabilitation companies are staffed with marketing specialists in addition to medical/vocational rehabilitation specialists. In these companies the marketing staff seeks out possible referral sources, describes the services offered, and collects information about the referring companies' needs. Using the needs information, the marketing people help to modify services to more closely meet the needs of potential or existing customers.

Some of the early adaptations which resulted from marketing efforts are today's standard services. As an example, many early companies got started by offering to review an insurance companies' files to identify appropriate candidates for rehabilitation services. Many companies now offer this service on an ongoing basis to all their regular customers as well as to potential customers. The rationale behind this service is that the rehabilitation agency helps to identify files which could show substantial savings through rehabilitation services. Once the file is reviewed, a supervisor has the opportunity to refer the case to the reviewer or to select another rehabilitation service provider (who obviously is not as convenient as the rehabilitation service provider who has just completed the review).

A second example of marketing technique used with insurance companies is a technique which has evolved into a regular service, the rehabilitation workshop. A member of the rehabilitation company conducts a workshop on the rehabilitation of insurance claimants for insurance company staff. In the workshop, the rehabilitation specialist may stress early identification of those needing rehabilitation services. The remainder of the workshop may focus on the rehabilitation company's success with their process for handling files. This is also an opportunity to highlight any special services provided by the rehabilitation company and to distinguish these from what other rehabilitation companies might offer. These workshops are often provided free or for a nominal fee. This type of service should not be confused with the training offered by a few rehabilitation companies whose stated goal is to assist their customers in developing better procedures internally. This is done to help the customer to work better with any rehabilitation company. In some instances, these companies are not even prepared to provide rehabilitation services for injured workers referred from insurance companies (or self-insured companies).

There are a variety of innovative marketing tools being used with insurance companies by rehabilitation service providers. Limited services, discounts for bulk referrals, and computerized summaries of a referral source's files might illustrate one company's unique qualities over those of another. A number of companies have also prepared movies, slide shows, or overhead slide presentations to more graphically demonstrate their special qualities.

Marketing is a critical component of successful private rehabilitation with the insurance industry, but it should not be the overwhelming emphasis of the company. In rare cases, a highly motivated marketing staff may bring in far more work than the existing staff can handle. It may also happen that overly zealous marketing personnel may accept too many older cases (late referrals), consequently overburdening the rehabilitation staff and resulting in poor results (Ostling, 1977).

The vast majority of rehabilitation companies are small. They can not afford the overhead of a staff member who does not perform work which can be billed. Consequently, most small companies market their services through their case handlers. The range of skills in the marketing area is very large. Some small companies have developed excellent working relationships with customers; others struggle to win and keep any company which will refer a file. The most successful companies employ counselors who promise only what they can deliver in the way of services, not referrals. This simple principle has proved to be a very profound one in the private rehabilitation sector.

Know the Facts

Rehabilitation professionals should know the law, the insurance company's style, and its method of providing rehabilitation services. It is also necessary to know the individual supervisor/adjuster's preferences. For instance, a benefit or service should never be suggested or promised to an injured worker until the referring claims person has been made aware of it. Some very embarrassing situations have developed because of such a failure to communicate. Counselors extend themselves too far when they promise benefits or services that they have failed to verify are actually available to an injured worker.

One dramatic example of this occurred in an eastern state in the late 1970s. A rehabilitation counselor working with a spinal cord injured worker developed a plan for the insurance company which included buying a home. The counselor had hoped to set up the injured worker in a business at this home. The law in this particular state allowed for the purchase of the home where no alternatives existed. The state itself had placed a cap on the amount of money that could be authorized for the purchase of a home. The counselor made only a minimal effort to explore alternatives and really did not know the law. He promised the injured worker a new home. As plans were being drawn up for the new home, the counselor forwarded his rehabilitation plan to the state workers' compensation agency. A copy of this plan was forwarded to the insurance company. The supervisor of the workers' compensation file had been unaware of the specific promises made by the counselor until he received this plan. The amount to be paid for the new home was well beyond what the supervisor could authorize or the state would require. In discussing this with the counselor, a dispute arose. The counselor was unable to understand why the insurance company would not agree to pay more than is required by law to help disabled persons.

A new rehabilitation counselor was then hired, and the case was quickly resolved, but the damage already done was substantial. The private rehabilitation industry received a black eye, and an injured worker was placed needlessly in the middle of a dispute. It is imperative that the specific requirements of the workers' compensation law be studied and understood by rehabilitation counselors who provide services for insurance companies.

Growing Pains

In California, a state which pioneered private sector rehabilitation during the 1970s, insurance companies were desperate to meet the mandates of the new workers' compensation law (Deneen & Hessellund, 1981). As each new private rehabilitation company was formed, their staff members found that getting files referred was relatively easy. They also found that low-paid, highly qualified rehabilitation counselors and registered nurses with some rehabilitation experience were eager to work in this enticing new field. A problem arose when, for example, Company A which provided outstanding services received more cases than its counselors, Carol and Tom, could handle. Before long, the marketing staff brought in so many new cases that additional staff members were hired. Carol and Tom could not work on all files, and so the casework quality plunged. Carol and Tom might have been given marketing responsibilities. Again service quality would plunge, and within a few months the company would lose many of its referral sources.

Another pattern disturbing to insurance companies in the early years of growth in California was the tendency among rehabilitation counselors/specialists to move frequently from one company to another or to leave a company to start their own companies. Although competition was welcomed by the users of the services, the changes often disrupted services to injured workers being served by the original company. In some instances embarrassing situations arose as the original company and the counselor or new employer struggled over possession of the files. Charges of violations of professionalism and of the code of ethics of rehabilitation counselors were made, but in most instances the issue was only resolved by a claim supervisor/adjuster who guessed what was best for the injured worker. These problems and others strained the credibility of all professional rehabilitation providers as the struggle for profits became more intense. Some rehabilitation service providers simply lost their sense of professionalism. Leaving without sufficient notice, taking cases from one's former employer, and speaking derogatorily about the former employer, all led outsiders to question the professionalism of rehabilitation people.

Their professionalism was further questioned when hints of "padding" bills with extra telephone charges and other services were first heard. It followed that the number of "billable hours" was also challenged and again the questions of padding was raised. Most private rehabilitation professionals hadn't even considered padding bills. The very few who succumbed to the temptation created an uneasy environment in which all rehabilitation service providers worked. Fortunately, the crisis passed with relatively few bills rejected and without a major scandal.

A Lesson Learned

Rehabilitation counselors who move from public or private nonprofit rehabilitation to the private-for-profit sector are often overwhelmed by the responsibilities and the apparent conflicts (Matkin & May, 1981). They find that in addition to providing traditional rehabilitation services, they must record and document their time. The counselor is often torn between a concern for the injured worker, the interests of the insurance company/self-insured company, and the interests of the rehabilitation company to achieve a profit.

It is important to keep in mind that although insurance companies pay out many billions of dollars in payments, they generally do so with strict controls. Rehabilitation bills may be reviewed by several staff members in some companies. In isolated instances the analysis of a bill may even involve interviewing those mentioned in the documentation of the bill.

It is also becoming more common for state workers' compensation agencies to monitor private rehabilitation service providers. There is a growing concern that insurance companies and self-insured companies may need assistance in these activities. California, Florida, and Minnesota have already taken steps to control who provides services. Several other states are considering implementing controls.

Summary

This chapter has introduced the reader to the insurance industry and explored its involvement in rehabilitation. Knowledge of the insurance industry is as important as rehabilitation knowledge for the private practitioner.

Insurance companies operate in many segments of society. They serve their policyholders and their stockholders (in the case of stock companies). They shape their practices to meet legal requirements, accepted insurance procedures, the demands of those buying the policies, and societal pressures for change (often to gain market shares).

Insurance companies produce a variety of products which require rehabilitation services to contain costs. Workers' compensation insurance is the line of insurance involving the largest number of rehabilitation referrals. No-fault automobile insurance, in some states, involves considerable rehabilitation services. The third line of insurance frequently involved in rehabilitation is long-term disability (LTD). The newest line of insurance to consider rehabilitation services is liability coverage. Although this is rarely seen, there is great potential for rehabilitation in liability cases.

Claim departments service the products sold by insurance companies. They are staffed by a variety of technicians including medical/vocational rehabilitation specialists. The great differences in staffing patterns and duties of staff people among insurance companies makes it imperative to learn about a company before attempting to provide services for it. There are a variety of ways in which a company may select and use outside rehabilitation services.

In 1981, five insurance companies collected more than 28% of all direct premiums for workers' compensation insurance. Liberty Mutual, Aetna Life and Casualty, The Travelers Insurance Companies, INA, and Hartford Insurance Group made up the top five. Although small companies may operate differently, learning about the operations of the five largest companies will provide insights into insurance company operations generally.

A number of insurance companies have their own subsidiaries. They have captured a significant percentage of the market nationwide, but in any specific location they may be less a factor. There does not appear to be any immediate threat that insurance company-owned rehabilitation companies will substantially increase their market share. Many fine rehabilitation companies (not owned by insurance companies) from Boston to San Francisco continue to grow and prosper. By producing quality results, both subsidiaries of insurance companies and privately owned rehabilitation companies will prosper.

Self-insurance as an adjunct or an alternative to insurance was discussed to make the reader aware of the trends in the market. This segment is an important one for those marketing insurance rehabilitation.

Marketing to any segment of the insurance market requires an understanding of the company, its products, and its needs. The relationship between those needs and the ability to provide services for them must also be explored.

There have been problems in the early years of private rehabilitation. The vast majority of private rehabilitation practitioners were not involved in this activity ten years ago. Despite the drastic change in their rehabilitation service responsibilities, most have adjusted very well.

Injured workers, the insurance industry, and the rehabilitation industry have benefited from insurance rehabilitation. Many more people will benefit in the years ahead as service delivery improves and referrals increase in response to that improvement.

References

Antwi, V. C-E Industrial Group, Kansas (Case No. 51, 479, December 6, 1980).

Best, A. M. *Best's executive data service: Property casualty insurance* (1981 edition). Oldwick, N.J.: A. M. Best Company, Inc., 1981.

Chamber of Commerce of the United States. *Analysis of workers' compensation laws*, Washington, D.C.: 1982.

Deneen, L. J., & Hessellund, T. A. *Vocational rehabilitation of the injured worker*. San Francisco: Rehabilitation Publications, 1981.

Eaton, M. W. Obstacles to the vocational rehabilitation of individuals receiving workers' compensation. *Journal of Rehabilitation*, 1979, *45*(2), 59–63.

Hatch, G. W. Jr. Resolution of workers' compensation claims. Video tape produced by The Travelers Insurance Company, 1979.

Larson, A. *Workmen's compensation for occupational injuries and death (Vol. 1)* New York: Matthew Bender, 1979.

Lewin, S. S., Ramseur, J. H., & Sink, J. M. The role of private rehabilitation: Founder, catalyst, competitor. *Journal of Rehabilitation*, 1979, *45*(3), 16–19.

Matkin, R. E. The certification dilemma in private rehabilitation. *Journal of Applied Rehabilitation Counseling*, 1981, *12*(1), 9–14.

Matkin, R. E., & May, R. V. Potential conflicts of interest in private rehabilitation: Identification and resolution. *Journal of Applied Rehabilitation Counseling*, 1981, *12*(1), 15–18.

Ostling, S. An insurance perspective of rehabilitation. A paper presented at the California Personnel and Guidance Association Annual Convention in San Francisco, Calif., February 19, 1977.

Sawyer, G. P. Private insurance company rehabilitation programming. A presentation made at the Southeastern Industrial Rehabilitation Institute, April 5–6, 1978.

Sawyer, G. P. Rehabilitation: A process in evolution. *IAIABC Journal*. August 1981, 13–17.

U.S. Department of Labor. *Dictionary of occupational titles, 4th edition*. Washington, D.C.: U.S. Government Printing Office, 1977.

U.S. Department of Labor. *Occupational outlook handbook, 1978–1979 edition*. Washington, D.C.: U.S. Government Printing Office, 1978.

Wales, J. T., & Ideson, H. A. *Claims law workers' compensation*. Basking Ridge, N.J.: American Educational Institute, 1977.

Waters, G. Florida workers' compensation rehabilitation program gets results. *Risk Management*, July 1981, 21–24.

4 The Rehabilitation Counselor as an Expert Witness in Personal-Injury Litigation

Ronald B. Harper

Introduction

During the past ten years, rehabilitation counselors have been called upon, with increasing frequency, to explain to civil courts of law just exactly what the impact of a serious injury has been on a person's employability. The purpose of this explanation, in the form of "expert witness testimony," is to provide the jury and/or judge with an objective account of how much the injured employee's future earning capacity has been affected, so that fair compensation can be awarded where liability for injury has been established.

Prior to the utilization of rehabilitation counselors to explain the financial impact of injury on earnings, attorneys attempted to accomplish this task with the help of physicians and economists. This approach never proved to be totally effective, since most physicians and economists did not have the background and expertise to testify on the qualifications, physical demands, and wages of some twenty thousand different occupations in the United States labor market. Accordingly, trial attorneys began to look around for a particular expertise to bridge this gap between the physician's statement of the physical and/or mental limitations brought about by the injury and the projected loss of earnings (and how they would be valued over a person's work-life expectancy).

The logical choice of a professional to fill this void of information was the rehabilitation counselor, who is charged with returning disabled individuals to appropriate employment in the labor market within the limitations placed upon them by their disability.

The purpose of this chapter is to present my experience as a vocational consultant and expert witness in matters of personal-injury litigation over the past ten years. Hopefully, this information will assist private sector rehabilitation counselors in performing the expert witness function more effectively—thus assisting injured parties in receiving fair and just compensation when warranted.

History of Vocational Expert Testimony

The use of persons trained and experienced in vocational counseling and job placement with disabled clients as expert witnesses in legal proceedings is rooted in the Social Security Administration's Disability Insurance Benefit Program. This program, which was legislated in 1954, provided for a freeze of benefits accrued to the date of disability. Later in 1956, legislation provided actual cash benefits upon establishment of proof of disability severe enough to prevent any type of employment.

Two levels of adjudication of disability status were established to be carried out by a designated state agency. They included the initial application for disability benefits, and, upon denial, the request for reconsideration of the claim. If claimants were denied on the second claim, they were given the opportunity to request a hearing before a Hearing Examiner of the Social Security Administration Bureau of Hearings and Appeals. (The position of Hearing Examiner has been since upgraded to Administrative Law Judge, and the agency is now known as the Office of Hearings and Appeals.)

Individuals who claimed they were too disabled to work and who were denied benefits by a Hearing Examiner were entitled to appeal this decision through the Federal Court System. In November, 1960, a decision issued by the United States Court of Appeals for the Second Circuit (*Kerner vs. Flemming*) held that a denial of disability benefits could not be sustained by a finding of mere theoretical ability to engage in substantial gainful activity. The court held that when it was clearly demonstrated that an individual was incapable of performing his or her regular occupation, the burden of proof fell upon the Social Security Administration to establish what other kind of work the individual could perform.

This decision established the "Kerner criteria." Thereafter, Hearing Examiners began citing published labor market information in their decisions, but eventually this approach was found to be inadequate by the courts. About 1962, the Social Security Administration (SSA) established criteria for vocational experts to be employed to offer direct testimony on the existence of appropriate jobs in the labor market. They established the following criteria for selecting these vocational experts:

A. Recent experience
   1. Rehabilitation counseling and/or placement, particularly with clients having prior work experience.
   2. The use of occupational materials developed for vocational counseling, including information about the requirements of jobs such as duties, skills, physical demands, working conditions, and occupationally significant charac-

teristics. A working knowledge of the *Dictionary of Occupational Titles* and its supplements is important.

3. The utilization of the concept of transferability of skills in terms of worker traits and functions.

B. Ability to observe and evaluate personal characteristics, educational, and vocational background.

C. Well-rounded, up-to-date knowledge of, and experience with, industrial and occupational trends and local labor market conditions.

Many claimants who requested a hearing before an SSA Hearing Examiner were represented by counsel, and these attorneys became quite familiar with the testimony of vocational experts and the value of the information they presented at the disability hearings. Because vocational experts were subject to cross-examination in these hearings, they became more skillful and utilized more careful documentation in presenting their testimony. It was only natural that the attorneys and the vocational experts would eventually form an alliance which would result in a more effective presentation of loss of earning capacity in personal-injury litigation. It was exactly the above sequence which brought me into this challenging work. Other than for the above historical perspective, the Social Security Disability Program will not be discussed in this chapter.

Qualifications of the Vocational Expert

I have already cited above the experiential criteria for vocational experts by the Social Security Administration's Office of Hearings and Appeals. These criteria do not specify any educational requirements, but I will tell you quite candidly—they are necessary. For this type of expert witness work, a professional with a doctorate is clearly preferred. Attorneys like to use expert witnesses whom they can address on the witness stand as "Doctor" because it clearly denotes that the professional has achieved the highest level of education in his or her field of endeavor. Most attorneys hope that jurors will be impressed with the high educational qualifications of their experts.

In my opinion, certification as a rehabilitation counselor and possession of a master's degree in rehabilitation counseling or one of the behavioral sciences along with several years of experience are minimal qualifications for courtroom testimony regarding the effect of injury on earning capacity.

However, please be aware that simply having excellent qualifications in the field as a rehabilitation counselor does not mean that those qualifications will readily be accepted by opposing counsel when you get to the courtroom. On several occasions I have seen opposing counsel make a motion to prevent me from testifying. Such motions have been made on the grounds that I was not qualified to testify on the issue of employability because my medical background was insufficient to understand the plaintiff's medical problems, or that my lack of training in economics prevented me from understanding the labor market, or the fact that I was not a licensed psychologist prevented me from understanding the plaintiff's emotional problems.

Usually, when such a motion is made, the judge will ask the opposing counsel to take you as a potential witness on *Voir Dire*. *Voir Dire* is a French phrase meaning "to speak the truth," but in legal terms it means the examination of the qualifications of a witness to testify on the subject at issue. You will be asked very penetrating questions about your knowledge of many subjects including some that are only remotely connected with disability or employment. Many of the questions will center around personal experiences with certain disabilities or occupations, such as whether you have actually watched a certain job being performed, or how many people you have counseled with a combination of a left-torn medial meniscus and an L4–L5 herniated nucleus pulposus, etc.

Voir Dire on your qualifications should never come as a surprise and should be always anticipated as a possibility. Each time you are preparing to testify, you should review your expertise about the plaintiff's disability, former occupations, and any proposed new occupations. If you are surprised by *Voir Dire* and become uncomfortable or defensive while the examination of your qualifications is taking place, the jury is going to notice and consider that behavior when they are weighing the worth of the rest of your testimony.

Types of Personal-Injury Litigation

The term personal-injury litigation simply means that an individual's person has been injured and that that person (the plaintiff) believes some other individual or entity (the defendant) is responsible for that injury. By the time you have been retained as a vocational expert, the courts will have established that sufficient grounds exist to put the matter into civil litigation.

Personal-injury litigation is usually conducted in the state superior court or federal district court systems. The majority of the litigation you will be involved in will take place in superior court. Personal-injury lawsuits that take place in federal court are usually those being tried under the Federal Employers Liability Act (injuries to seamen or fishermen) or, in certain cases, those wherein the defendant company is operating in many states and headquartered in another state. Of course, suits against the United States Government always take place in the Federal Court System.

Please note that we are not talking about workers' compensation for an injury on the job. For example, some personal injuries may also be industrial injuries, but the defendant being sued is usually not the employer, but rather a third party such as the manufacturer of a machine that has malfunctioned or another company operating a vehicle on the premises. Workers' compensation is a completely different topic, and it will not be addressed in this chapter.

Some examples of personal injury most often litigated include the following:

1. Injuries caused by malfunctioning machinery or equipment.
2. Injuries caused by disregard of safety regulations or obvious negligence in industrial settings.
3. Injuries caused by motor vehicle accidents that are due to negligent drivers.
4. Injuries caused by faulty medical equipment or medical malpractice.
5. Injuries caused by firearms and batons used negligently by law enforcement personnel.
6. Injuries of employees of railroads in the course of their work.
7. Injuries of commercial fishermen and seamen in commercial shipping in the course of their work.

As a vocational expert, you may be approached by either the plaintiff's attorney or the defendant's attorney to assess the impact of personal injury on future earning potential regarding any of the above types of litigated injuries.

Limitations of the Rehabilitation Counselor's Expertise as a Vocational Witness

The function of the rehabilitation counselor in personal-injury litigation is to offer an opinion on the impact of the injury on the individual's future earning capacity. In other words, you are being asked to estimate in dollars and cents what an individual can earn or be trained to earn after their injury or if they are employable at all. This is actually *all* you are being asked to do, and it is very important that you do only that and no more or no less.

You are not called into these matters to give a psychological diagnosis or prognosis. For example, you are not being asked to predict economic conditions over the next twenty years. It is very important that you recognize the boundaries of your expertise and that you inform the attorneys who seek your opinion on employability exactly what constitutes the boundaries of your profession. I have often been called on to assess employability and then also have been asked to make an economic prediction of work-life expectancy, rates of inflation, interest rates, and such by attorneys who want a two-for-one witness. I always tell them that I am not an economist, and I will not attempt to impersonate one on the witness stand.

You must remember that when you are on a witness stand and you stray out of your field and your qualifications to testify in some peripheral area, you may be challenged seriously. This may detract from your earlier testimony when you were qualified to give opinions. In other words, by getting out of your field, you risk losing your credibility with the court altogether and negate what legitimate information you have already offered. Therefore, stick to vocational rehabilitation, which is your professional field of experience.

In view of what I have just stated, when you are approached by either the plaintiff or defense attorney to give an opinion on an injured party's employability, make sure you and the attorney are very clear on the referral question. Both of you should know why you are being consulted and exactly what type of opinion you are to provide, when it is to be provided, and in what form it will be provided – whether verbal or written. I usually ask the attorney to put this request in writing so there will be no misunderstanding in what is expected of me in the way of a professional opinion.

In most cases of personal-injury litigation, both sides must list their potential expert witnesses with the court between thirty and sixty days before trial. Therefore, the clarification of your professional role should take place before you allow your name to be submitted, to avoid misunderstanding or embarrassment to you and the attorney.

Vocational Evaluation of the Injured Plaintiff

The techniques you use to vocationally evaluate the injured plaintiff may vary somewhat depending on whether you are working for the plaintiff attorney or the defense attorney. This variation pertains mainly to evaluating the plaintiff on behalf of the defendant. It is not always easy to get permission to evaluate the plaintiff for a defense attorney in the same way you would normally perform a vocational evaluation for the plaintiff's own attorney. If the plaintiff's attorney does not agree to the evaluation, the defense attorney must seek a court order to compel the plaintiff to submit to the vocational evaluation. This can be done in Federal Court, but in state courts it may be more difficult.

In the state of California, where I practice, it is almost impossible to vocationally evaluate a plaintiff for a defendant in a superior court case unless the plaintiff agrees to the evaluation. This situation is the result of a 1979 California Court of Appeals decision known as *Browne vs. Superior Court*. In this decision the court ruled that a plaintiff cannot be compelled under discovery rules to submit to a physical examination by a vocational rehabilitation counselor who is not also a "licensed physician." Although the courts have been liberal in allowing "discovery" in the form of defense-ordered medical examinations, to avoid surprise they chose not to allow such non-medical discovery, stating that it overstepped the intent of the legislature. Therefore, when you find yourself in this situation, you must rely on records of others to offer an opinion, and even when you do this, you are quite vulnerable to cross-examination in depositions or in court. You must examine all of the medical reports, personnel records, reports of other rehabilitation agencies, and depositions of physicians, plaintiffs, and rehabilitation experts. If it is possible, you should listen to the plaintiff's experts testify before you do.

When conducting a vocational evaluation on behalf of an injured plaintiff or with the plaintiff's permission for the defense, the process is much the same as you would use in your regular rehabilitation counseling practice. The evaluation should consist of the following steps:

1. Acquisition and review of all available documentary information such as medical reports, personnel records, high-school and college transcripts, depositions of the plaintiff, as well as other medical and vocational experts.
2. A comprehensive interview to gather information on educational background, employment history, functional limitations resulting from the injury, and past attempts at vocational rehabilitation.
3. Administration of intelligence, academic achievement, dexterity, aptitude, and vocational interest tests.
4. Analysis of the available information and the formation of an opinion as to whether the plaintiff is employable or can be employable with training, and if so at what type of work. Estimation of availability and level of financial compensation for the proposed employment.

I cannot stress strongly enough the need for gathering accurate, verified information. You must constantly bear in mind that any opinion you render either verbally or in written form may well be subject to rigorous cross examination at some point in the future. If you are testifying in court and are presented with new information regarding a plaintiff's prison record, evidence of being disciplined on a job, substance abuse, misrepresentation of types of work or level of salary, etc., you may find it quite embarrassing, and the jury will start to question other information the plaintiff has provided you. Therefore, it is very important that you document all of your information as thoroughly as possible. For example, always get school records if they are available to compare results of standardized school testing with your own test results. Do the same with employment records so if you find discrepancies in length of employment or salary earned, you can resolve them before rendering a vocational opinion.

One of the most important concepts to remember in performing evaluations of employability in personal-injury litigation is that you must approach each situation with an open mind and avoid prejudging a plaintiff until you have gathered all of the information. Most of the time personal-injury evaluations do not result in a nice, neat percentage like a workers' compensation schedule rating of a disability. I will give two examples to illustrate my point.

A few years ago I was asked to evaluate a 55-year-old man who had lost part of his little finger at the middle point on his right major hand due to a crush injury while working as a railroad track laborer. The California schedule for rating industrial injuries would rate this injury at 4% disability. When I testified in the lawsuit, I explained to the court that the man spoke only Spanish but could neither read nor write the Spanish language. He had grown up in Mexico and never attended any type of school. Testing results indicated that he had a nonverbal I.Q. of about 80. Medical reports confirmed that there were several neuromas in the stump of the finger, and that when the stump was bumped even slightly, the pain radiated up to the shoulder due to an inflamed nerve pathway.

The result was that every time the man's finger was bumped, even with gloves on, the man's arm felt like it was being torn off. Examining physicians agreed that the man's right major arm and hand were essentially useless because of this condition. The man had only performed unskilled heavy manual labor during his working lifetime and was untrainable for any type of work that did not require repetitive use of his major arm and hand. Accordingly, he had to be considered 100% disabled and was given a sizable award by the jury.

In another instance I was asked to evaluate a 20-year-old young man who had suffered a spinal cord injury in an automobile accident which resulted in paraplegia. He was attending a local university, and psychological testing revealed that he had an I.Q. of 127 in the superior range of intelligence. He was planning to major in accounting, and his career goal was to become a CPA. The industrial injury rating schedule would have rated him as 100% disabled because of his paralysis. However, his employment prospects were certainly far better than the laborer mentioned above who lost part of a finger.

My point is simply that there is no easy system or formula for performing these evaluations. You have to take them one at a time and weigh all of the factors before reaching a conclusion. Each plaintiff is a unique individual and will require an individualized evaluation. The plaintiff's level of employability may well depend as much on mental capacity, educational, and vocational background as much as it does on the severity of the injury.

Although I rarely see out-and-out malingering (which I define as the pretense of incapacity for financial gain), I recognize that the plaintiff wishes to present their situation to their best advantage with regard to their quest for compensation. Accordingly, they may omit, or be reluctant to volunteer, certain information which you may consider quite important. This may occur at an almost unconscious level, so it is your responsibility to dig out all of the information that would have an influence on employability and verify it.

Your findings may also be used as a foundation for the testimony of an economist as an expert witness on long-term economic loss throughout the work-life expectancy of the plaintiff. So if your information is compromised, the economist who comes behind you is also in trouble.

Presentation of Opinion on Employability through Reports or Depositions

After an opinion on an injured plaintiff's employability has been formulated, it may be presented to the referring attorney either verbally or in the form of a report. Unless there is a reasonable opportunity to settle the matter, many attorneys prefer a verbal report, so they do not have to turn over a written report to opposing counsel during the discovery period. When opposing counsel receives such a report, they usually give it to their own vocational expert to be researched and refuted.

If a written report is requested, it should not be lengthy, since it may go into evidence and the jury, opposing counsel and the judge, etc., already have voluminous medical records, personnel records, and reports from other experts to review. The report should cover educational background, employment history, functional limitations as presented by treating and examining physicians and psychologists, results of psychological tests, and a final section summarizing your conclusions.

The discussion section of your report should explain why the individual's injury prevents him/her from physically and/or mentally performing a former occupation. You should then explain why the individual is unemployable, if this is the case. If there are other jobs the person can perform or be trained to perform, give specific examples of what they are and relate them to the plaintiff's test performance and physical limitations. You should then give salary ranges for these proposed occupations and cite your salary information sources. A statement on the current salary range of the plaintiff's former occupations is also helpful.

When a formal vocational report has not been prepared and submitted, many times opposing counsel will subpoena you for a deposition in order to find out what you are going to say in court, if the case goes to trial. This is perfectly legal during the discovery period prior to the beginning of trial.

A deposition is a process whereby you are placed under oath by a certified court stenographer and cross-examined by opposing counsel on your vocational opinion and your reasons for reaching that opinion. Your entire testimony is recorded and transcribed and put into a booklet form. After the transcription, you are given an opportunity to proofread the transcript of your testimony and correct any statements you did not mean to make or which did not reflect your intended meaning.

In some ways, giving a deposition is more difficult than testimony in court because there is not a judge present to rule on objections. You have to try to answer every question unless instructed not to answer by your retaining counsel, which seldom happens. You will hear your retaining counsel object to many questions, but in the absence of a judge, you still have to try to answer them, no matter how irrelevant or distant from your field they may be. Be sure to obtain and reread a copy of your deposition before you go to court, because you certainly want to be consistent in what you say. If you have said one thing in a deposition and another in court, opposing counsel will be sure to let you know it and use it to impeach your testimony before the court. It is my practice, prior to trial, to review the deposition and make notes on all questions for which I thought my answers were weak or for which I did not have the information requested. I then take steps to shore up those answers and locate the needed information. Usually, when an attorney finds a weak area in a deposition, he or she will return to that area in courtroom cross-examinations. Therefore, never discount the value of a deposition in the preparation of courtroom testimony.

Courtroom Testimony

After the report has been submitted, the deposition taken, and all attempts to settle the case have been exhausted, the matter on which you have been retained will go to trial, and you will be called to testify on your vocational opinion.

It is extremely important that you spend some time with your retaining attorney in the preparation of testimony. Attorneys vary in their attitude toward how this should be done. Some of them will want to come to your office and spend two hours going over every detail of your qualifications, findings, and conclusions. Others will want to prepare testimony during a fifteen-minute court recess. The former may be too much time, the latter certainly too little time. The important thing to remember is that the attorney's questions have to elicit the salient details of your findings about the client's vocational abilities and the availability and level of compensation of proposed residual employment. In cases of plaintiffs found to be unemployable, the details of your reasons for such a finding have to be brought out clearly.

I often prepare a brief outline of questions that will best bring out the information gathered and the vocational opinion being presented. The following is an example:

1. Of what did your evaluation consist?
2. Please summarize the information gathered in the interview.
3. Please summarize the vocational testing results.
4. Please tell us what documents (medical reports, school transcripts, personnel records, etc.) you have reviewed regarding the plaintiff.
5. Based on all of the information you have obtained from your evaluation and have reviewed from other sources, do you have an opinion regarding the plaintiff's current level of employability? Training potential for future employability?
6. Do you have any comment on employers' attitudes on hiring disabled job applicants?

It is that simple. The direct testimony should seldom involve more than those six questions. However, it is not always an easy matter to confine your retaining attorney to six questions. If the testimony is going well, there are no objections, and the jury is attentive, the attorney may decide to throw in some additional questions like: Hasn't it been your experience that no employer will hire a person who has had a back injury? If you answer that question "yes," you are probably committing perjury, and if you answer "no," you are indicating to the jury that the attorney is obviously trying to influence your testimony. This type of situation should be anticipated and avoided. Tell the attorney in no uncertain terms that he is not to stray from the agreed questions because most of the time the result will not be good. Be firm on this issue.

When appearing in court, dress conservatively. This admonition has nothing to do with your individual taste in clothes. You are there to present information that you want to be heard and comprehended by a jury. Therefore, your appearance should do nothing to distract their attention from what you are saying to them. Do not be concerned about being a little nervous when you sit down, as the jury expects it. By the time you testify, they will have heard several witnesses and have learned that they are all nervous. If you aren't a little nervous and appear too self-confident, they probably won't trust you anyway. After testifying over two hundred times in court, I never fail to feel a few butterflies in my stomach just prior to sitting in the witness stand.

In this entire process, undergoing cross-examination is the most stressful segment. There is no easy way to prepare you for this exercise. It covers a broad range of experiences from tepid to devastating. All I can tell you is to listen to the questions *very* carefully, and if you don't understand the question, say so and ask for clarification. Some of the questions will be totally incomprehensible, and you should not even attempt a response to them. Do not speculate or go beyond the information you have, because if you do, you are sure to get into trouble.

Be aware in advance that you will be asked on most occasions at the beginning of cross-examination about how many times you have appeared in court for plaintiff or defense attorneys and how much you are charging for your services. Often the cross-examiner will try to portray you as a professional witness who makes a living by going to court and testifying every day for high fees and as a person who will offer any opinion desired if paid to do so. Please do not take this as a personal attack or as evidence that the opposing counsel "just doesn't like you." The attorneys are just doing their job, and the attorney who hired you probably has or will do the same thing to the opposing witnesses. An attorney who responds to you in this way may call you to work on one of his cases the following week! Probably the most useful advice I can give you on the subject of cross-examination is to be clear in your own mind as to where your responsibility in the courtroom as an expert witness begins and ends. You are there to offer an opinion on what type of employment an injured person can or cannot perform and to give your reasons for that opinion. You are not there to help the retaining attorney try the case, and you are not there as a plaintiff advocate or critic. You are not responsible for the circumstances behind the information you have been given to work with, and you have no obligation to defend the plaintiff against legitimate criticism or aid and abet illegitimate charges against her or him. Just answer the questions as truthfully and unemotionally as possible, and you will successfully survive the experience. Do not be afraid to say "I don't know"; it is no sin and certainly helps the jury to understand that you are just an ordinary person who doesn't know everything. Remember, thorough, careful preparation and a well-organized file (which opposing counsel will probably review before cross-examination) cut down the anxiety.

Fees

Knowing what to charge for your services is always a dilemma. I have tried various fee schedules and combinations of hourly rates and half-day block rates, etc. Invariably, when I used a block-fee system of charging two hundred and fifty dollars or three hundred dollars for a half-day for courtroom testimony, I would experience some awkward moments on the witness stand. For example, opposing counsel would ask: "Dr. Harper, what are you charging for your appearance here today?" If my answer was three hundred dollars, the attorney might ask if that in reality constituted a rate of three hundred dollars per hour since it did not appear that my testimony would take any longer than that, and wasn't three hundred dollars an hour certainly more lucrative than working as a counselor for some agency. Get the point?

Accordingly, about two years ago, I went to an hourly rate for every service I perform. I keep that hourly rate in the competitive range with other vocational, economic, psychological, and engineering experts. It seems to go down a little easier to be able to say I am charging eighty-five dollars per hour, since the attorney asking you knows he is charging one hundred dollars per hour for being there himself. If pressed on fees, I will occasionally slip in a comment about my hourly rate being less than that charged by most attorneys.

In a tight cash-poor economy such as now exists, collecting fees can be a persistent and frustrating problem. Many attorneys, especially sole practitioners or partners in small firms, do not have a lot of financial resources available to pay for case preparation, since they accept most of these cases on the contingency that they will receive a percentage of any settlement or award.

A few years ago, after discovering that I had some twenty thousand dollars out in unpaid receivable fees, I decided that my policy of trusting plaintiff attorneys to pay my fees in a timely fashion deserved some serious reexamination (defense attorneys are no major problem since your fees are paid by the liability insurance carrier; you may wait six weeks, but you will be paid). I decided at that point to go to a monetary retainer system. If a plaintiff attorney wishes a written report, I ask for a retainer covering the cost of seven hours of services in advance. This amounts to five hours for an evaluation and two hours to analyze the information and write the report. The attorney is forewarned of the possibility of overrunning that time frame, and the attorney is billed for the balance. I ask for five hours in advance if only a verbal report is requested.

I usually trust them for the testimony fees unless they have a poor payment history with me, and then I ask for an advance payment of a couple of hours. This system, of course, does not eliminate the collection problem. Even when you trust them the first time, you may find that they will lose the case on a liability issue, meaning they could not prove that the injury was caused by the entity being sued. The result of that outcome is that they have to pay the trial expenses out of their own pocket, which may be empty.

After six months, I file against them in small claims court, and I can truthfully say that in the few instances where I have had to file, I have never had to appear in court. The debt was always paid prior to the trial. When faced with the embarrassing prospect of having to appear in court for non-payment of a debt, attorneys always seem to find a way to get the money they owe to you.

To avoid any later misunderstanding or confusion, always make it very clear in the beginning what your fee structure is and that you expect to be paid promptly after services are rendered. You may be offered a chance to wait for your fee until the trial is concluded and a successful verdict is rendered and told that you will then be paid much more than your regular fee. Never accept such arrangements, because if you do and it is somehow discovered, your credibility in the legal community will be seriously damaged. It will be said that your testimony was certainly affected by the fact that you stood to gain more financially from a successful outcome of the case.

Information Resources

In order to function successfully as a vocational expert in personal-injury litigation, you must have a great deal of current occupational and related information at your fingertips. Be prepared to invest a great deal of time and several hundred dollars in building your resource library. Here is a list of the minimal essential information you will need:

1. *Dictionary of Occupational Titles, 4th Edition*, 1977.
2. *Selected Characteristics of Occupations Defined in the D.O.T.*, 1981.
3. Current wage and salary surveys.
4. Current *Occupational Outlook Handbook*.
5. Several current textbooks on psychological testing.
6. Research information on employer attitudes toward hiring disabled persons.
7. A good medical dictionary.
8. *The Merck Manual of Diagnosis and Therapy*.
9. Copies of all state and federal regulations pertaining to licensure or certification in government-regulated occupations.
10. *The Physician's Desk Reference*, current edition.
11. Copies of all federal regulations pertaining to the Rehabilitation Act of 1973 (500 to 504 series).
12. A list of legal experts in other fields of expertise, especially psy-

chology and economics and vocational experts throughout the United States.

13. Subscriptions to the *Journal of Rehabilitation*, *Personnel and Guidance Journal*, *Occupational Outlook Quarterly*, and *Rehabilitation Psychology*.
14. *Diagnostic and Statistical Manual of Mental Disorders, Third Edition*, 1980.

In addition to the above, I read two daily newspapers, the *Wall Street Journal*, the local legal newspaper, the state weekly insurance news magazine, the *Personnel Administrator*, and a news magazine about the disabled. I am constantly clipping articles on labor, industry, medicine, and the handicapped to be placed in over one hundred different topical files. Remember, as a consultant, a major part of your job is to provide up-to-date accurate information and to do that you have to read a lot of material.

Conclusion

In the previous pages, I have tried to bring you an overview of how a rehabilitation counselor functions as a valuable source of expertise in the area of personal-injury litigation.

One of the reasons I have finally taken the time to do this is because I am very proud of the profession of rehabilitation counseling, a profession in which I have functioned for over twenty years. Rehabilitation counselors have provided a valuable service to the disabled citizens of the United States for nearly sixty years and assisted countless thousands in returning to meaningful employment in our society. In learning how to do that, rehabilitation counselors have become experts in many vocational areas. The legal profession has grown to respect that expertise and is now willing to pay for it.

5 Working as a Rehabilitationist in Business Organizations

Paul Scher

Introduction

The purpose of this chapter is to discuss the role of the rehabilitation counselor in private industry. These practitioners work for organizations whose mission is the production of goods or the sale of services other than counseling. The existence of a counseling service is provided as a staff function for the purpose of maintaining psychological well-being and effective morale within the workforce. Counseling services are used not only by some of the Fortune 500 companies but also by a variety of smaller firms who contract out for counseling services.

Rehabilitation practitioners are employed by industry in order to assist their organizations to meet four goals. These goals are

1. A reduction in the overall cost of managing people by reducing the number of people-caused problems.
2. The reduction and prevention of illnesses caused by stress and substance abuse.
3. The treatment of physical and mental illness as an alternative to termination.
4. The provision of career guidance and retirement counseling for work effectiveness.

It is important that a rationale for using counseling services as a human resources management tool be understood. In this way, specific examples of company programs can be comprehended within a context of applied counseling theory and practice.

Rehabilitation Counseling as a Human Resources Management Tool

Counseling functions consist in helping people to meet problems, make decisions, and do a better job of progressing through life. Rehabilitation counseling then is a dispenser of services designed to help an impaired person overcome the handicap caused by a disability. But such a tool is equally appropriate for assisting employed persons, be they disabled or not, to retain their equilibrium so as to cope with life's challenges. The employer becomes interested in the capacity of the worker to meet adequately these challenges when failure to do so results in deteriorating or unacceptable work performance.

Employees are the most important resource of any business. Without them, nothing is accomplished. The physical and mental well-being of the employee affect the quantity and quality of work produced. The recognition of this fact on the part of business is resulting in the expansion of the traditional personnel function to include a broader understanding of the needs of the entire person. Therefore, counseling which encompasses a recognition of the individual's needs is transferable from the office of the psychologist to a corner of confidentiality in the workplace. Thus, the recognition of individual versatility necessitates a holistic approach in respect to the management of people.

Human resources management shows a concern for the health and well-being of employees. This recognition is reflected in the praise of success and the correction of poor performance. But these functions are carried out in the spirit of concern for the growth, development, and psychological stability of the employee.

The United States Clearing House for Mental Health Education reports that industry has had a $17-billion annual reduction in its productive capacity because of stress-induced mental dysfunctions (Appelbaum, 1980). Losses due to stress-induced physical illness are doubtless even greater. It is obvious that the effects of excessive stress are not only counterproductive but very costly in terms of employee hospital plans, long-term disability insurance coverage, and unnecessary early retirement. Personnel costs are increasing at an alarming rate. Salaries have increased 100% in the past 11 years. One-fourth of an employee's payroll was made up of the cost of fringe benefits in 1977. The U.S. Chamber of Commerce estimated that fringe benefits made up 40% of the payroll in 1980 (Martin, 1980). The way to reduce these costs involves recognizing individual needs while at the same time rewarding good performance and correcting poor performance. Supervisors learn to do this within a framework of concern for the individual.

Personnel administration practiced within a framework of human resources management still deals with manpower problems, salary administration, human resources planning, equal opportunity, affirmative action, and benefits administration. In an atmosphere of concern, industrial relations are comfortable and labor negotiations are easier (Compshare brochure). Personnel practices within such a framework can be characterized by tendencies like these:

1. Turning away from a view of people as essentially bad to a view of people as basically good.
2. Avoiding negative evaluation and confirming the person as a human being.
3. Moving away from seeing individuals as fixed and toward seeing them as a process.
4. Moving away from resisting the reality of individual differences and toward utilizing these differences.
5. Moving away from utilizing an individual primarily with reference to job descriptions and toward utilizing the individual as a whole person.
6. Moving away from primarily placing emphasis on competition and toward a greater emphasis on collaboration. (Applebaum & Davis, 1980).

With such changes in orientation, the organization can help people make decisions and cope with life's stresses. So can the counselor. So can the rehabilitation practitioner. Counseling serves as a tool for regulating the process of helping employees do a better job. By using this tool, the company increases its cost effectiveness.

How Cost-Effective?

In 1980, 37 states contained provisions in the workers' compensation laws which make rehabilitation services at the employer's expense available to the injured worker. International Rehabilitation Associates, the largest private rehabilitation firm with offices in the United States, Canada, and Australia, analyzed almost 3,000 cases. Based upon an analysis of 13,392 workers' compensation cases in 1979, it was determined that the average cost of rehabilitation to the insurer was $1,019. Each case was open for an average of 9.6 months. The average return on every rehabilitation dollar spent was $12.28. Of vocational plans put into effect, 90% of the disabled clients returned to work (Welch, 1979).

An employee assistance program makes counseling services available on a voluntary basis for personal or job-related problems. The types of problems brought to the employee assistance counselor run the gamut of social concerns. They include stress-related matters caused by insufficient training or ambiguous goals, poor work performance because of lack of communication, stress caused by a variety of home problems, addiction to alcohol or other substances, and financial strain.

A search of the literature (conducted by the insurance industry) has revealed that the following results can be expected after employee assistance programs have been established:

A 20% reduction in lost man hours.

A 61% reduction in the cost of medical benefits.

A 74% reduction in the number of disciplinary actions.

A rehabilitation recovery rate of between 65% and 85% of troubled employees (Rose, n.d.).

What a potential savings in the cost of employee maintenance!

It can be seen that employee assistance programs use rehabilitation counseling as a tool to adjust the degree of harmony within the workplace. It is also obvious that industry is not adopting counseling services for philanthropic purposes. While it is true that work expectation today includes an atmosphere conducive to the "good life," a company can meet this expectation and at the same time reduce in part those expenses which are incurred if capable employees fail to be rehabilitated and if troubled employees are allowed to receive a benefit or retire early. Rehabilitation becomes an important management tool in a program designed to conserve and maximize the effectiveness of its most precious resource, its employees.

Examples of Rehabilitation Programs in Industry

It was pointed out that counseling services are used within industry for rehabilitating injured workers, administrating employee assistance programs, and operating career guidance centers. There are enough companies with such programs to write a text solely on these activities. Among those companies which utilize counseling services, a few have been selected to illustrate a variety of structures and approaches to service delivery.

3M Company

The St. Paul-based 3M Company employs approximately 55,000 individuals. Its rehabilitation services program is located within its human resources organization. The company uses the terms "sector" to denote profit-making centers and "organization" to denote what is usually thought of as a staff-support function. This is important because industry today is preoccupied with a felt need to reorganize its activities in such a way as to accommodate a more holistic approach to the variety of functions necessary for success.

The program is staffed by a rehabilitation services supervisor and a placement specialist. The supervisor holds an M.A. in psychology and is licensed to practice by the state of Minnesota. He also is a Certified Rehabilitation Counselor (C.R.C.) and a Q.R.C., Qualified Rehabilitation Counselor, as required by the licensure law in Minnesota. The responsibilities of the supervisors are nationwide. At any one time they have a case load of approximately 600 to manage. These individuals represent employees injured on the job, those who have developed disabilities, and some new employees with handicaps newly entering the labor market. It is necessary to contract out for services because of the wide distribution of 3M facilities. Yet, the supervisor is responsible for overall plan development and execution.

The company believes that the practice of industrial rehabilitation counseling involves more than being skilled as a psychologist and a rehabilitation practitioner: it is also necessary to know the structure of the company thoroughly. A knowledge of collective bargaining and negotiation procedures are essential. In addition to a familiarity with company and federal benefits, a deep understanding of disincentives to work is required in dealing with the many problems that the disabled employees and their families face. Each individual must be helped on a case-by-case basis, and resources have to be located that can meet the particular needs of the client, according to 3M. As the rehabilitation plan is developed, recommendations must be submitted to management for its approval. Attitudes of supervisors and co-workers must be dealt with. The counselor must be aware of the family configuration in every case.

The rehabilitation unit also advises the company in respect to meeting affirmative action requirements regarding the recruitment, placement, training, and advancement of qualified handicapped workers. A firm is fortunate to have a rehabilitation service which can assist in this activity. The company operates a "handivan," which accommodates wheelchairs. A "van pool" system is also maintained, helping both disabled and nondisabled employees get to and from work. The company also operates an employee assistance program for employees with alcohol abuse problems. A personnel development section assists with career guidance for 3M's employees. Thus, this organization has for some time realized the conserving power of rehabilitation as a management resource component.

Control Data Corporation

Control Data in Minneapolis employs 57,000 people. At any given time, 1 to 3% are on medical leave, or about 1,000 people. Of these, 30–40% require rehabilitation intervention. At Control Data, rehabilitation services are provided by the Employee Advisory Resource, their employee assistance program. Approximately 800 new cases are seen each month in the Minneapolis and Baltimore facilities. The service is trusted, for it maintains a high degree of confidentiality.

The program is organized under the Vice President of Human Resources. It is run by a general manager. The manager has a background in business and a masters degree in counseling psychology. The staff consists of 25 people, and consultants are utilized. There are counselors on staff who specialize in alcohol dependency. One individual holds a masters degree in counseling psychology. Twenty are based in Minneapolis while five reside in Baltimore. Most of the referrals are made by telephone. A good deal of counseling is done by telephone, and it may include simply instructing managers or employees in trouble how to find appropriate assistance. The program is voluntary, but managers are trained to relate poor performance to job requirements and to advise that counseling be sought when appropriate. Both clinics operate 24 hours a day. Counseling services are provided not only to the employee but to the employee's family, particularly in the case of the industrially injured. Those with industrial injuries, multiple sclerosis, cardiovascular accidents (CVAs), or spinal cord injuries all require and obtain competent rehabilitation services. When necessary, rehabilitation vendors are employed but are supervised by one of the Control Data counseling staff. At remote locations counseling staff is not available. In these cases, the staff will advise the employee how to seek appropriate counseling or medical care and then follow up to be sure that the individual has procured these services.

The program has dealt with almost every human concern. An employee who developed epilepsy was able to retain his job after the counseling staff pointed out to the supervisor that his lapses of attentiveness were not due to lack of interest but rather to epilepsy.

Ken Anderson (1980), program founder, reported that $350,000 was saved in direct costs the first year. An additional half million was saved in indirect costs. Direct savings include compensation not paid because the employee returned to work, reduced hospital stay, elimination of the need for LTD, and the financial advantages of paying salary instead of benefits. Indirect savings include litigation not needed, retraining that was avoided, and families able to remain independent. Eligibility for using the service is not limited to those who are injured on the job. Family members are treated for school problems, stress, marital difficulty—the entire range of human concerns. Control Data feels that its Employee Advisory Resource is well worth the cost.

Xerox Corporation

The Xerox Corporation, whose president was Chairman of the U.S. Committee for the International Year of Disabled Persons, is in the process of developing an internal rehabilitation program. The versatility of models within private industry is illustrated by the fact that rehabilitation intern Joan Hoeffel (1979) was able to demonstrate at Xerox that group counseling is an effective, efficient, and economical form of rehabilitating industrial employees who suffer from chronic pain. The experiment involved 32 employees with lower back problems. They were divided into two groups, one of which received individual counseling. The remainder received group counseling. All worked for Xerox. All were entitled to the same employee benefits. All of them felt isolated and anxious and experienced muscle tension and family difficulties. Time at work lost by members of the group ranged from 8 to 345 weeks.

Thirty-seven percent of those receiving individual therapy returned to work compared to 45% of those receiving group therapy. It was concluded that there are advantages to the group process in rehabilitating chronic pain patients. The synergy of the group seems to accelerate learning, positive attitudes, and behaviors which in turn promote heightened self-esteem and increased ability to cope with chronic pain. The fact that treatment is sponsored by the corporation also contributes to building a positive attitude in the employee.

For our purposes, the study is not as important as the illustration that it provides. A rehabilitation program run by well trained and responsible personnel can make a valuable contribution to the stability of the company's work force. The dollars saved by the company that would have been spent in ongoing employee benefits are obviously significant.

Sears, Roebuck and Company

Sears employs slightly under 320,000 employees nationally. The Handicapped Program is located in the Equal Opportunity section managed by the Director of Employee Relations and Equal Opportunity, who is responsible to the Vice President of Personnel and Employee Relations. The author of this chapter manages the company's handicapped program.

A policy directive contained in the Sear's Personnel Manual authorizes the establishment of employee assistance programs, and rehabilitation terminology is used in several places in respect to company health and long-term disability plans.

The Handicapped Program is based on affirmative action. It involves the continuous evaluation of a Selective Placement Manual, advises employee benefits policymakers regarding appropriate rehabilitation policy, and undertakes a variety of public service activities designed to familiarize the commercial community with the capabilities of disabled workers.

A rehabilitation service is established within the legal department in Sears Western Territory to service workers' compensation claims. There, an experienced personnel worker and an assistant deal with the claims of injured workers and assist them and their families to develop and execute rehabilitation plans. Rehabilitation plans prepared by this staff are accepted by the California Rehabilitation Bureau. Sears has experienced a high rate of success in returning these employees to jobs. All four legal departments are gaining experience in the use of industrial rehabilitation personnel.

Under Sears' broad policy, four model employee assistance programs function. A troubled-employee hotline in the Western Territory operates out of Alhambra, California. In three years it has assisted over 300 employees in nine western states.

Sears Tower in Chicago operates an alcoholism control program. Its recovery rate (recovery defined as staying sober for a year or longer) has reached 80%. A consultant is used who specializes in alcohol dependency. His office is easily accessible, located in the Medical Department in such a way that clients can enter discreetly. The counselor also deals with other personal problems and refers employees to an appropriate agency if they are beyond his scope of practice.

Sears units in Miami participate with neighbors in the business community in an employee assistance program. Periodically, information is given to supervisors and employees regarding the availability of services, how to make a referral, and how to detect that an individual is getting into difficulty. In short, a policy exists permitting any Sears territory, group, or unit to establish an employee assistance program using available resources in the community. This policy permits the flexibility required in a company as large as Sears. The establishment of a greater number of employee assistance programs is planned.

J. C. Penney

J. C. Penney (Egdahl & Walsh, 1980) operates a counseling program attached to a special health services section under the supervision of the medical director in New York. The organization has 185,000 employees, who are based across the country. The chief counselor is trained in the area of alcoholism control, but his services are available to help employees whose problems interface with their work performance for any reason. This person is also responsible for maintaining a hotline by which managers can be instructed on how to find appropriate resources for a troubled employee and how to confront their poor work performance with the suggestion that they seek counseling in preference to termination. Some specialized training is given to managers regarding confrontation techniques. At J. C. Penney, employees are not confronted on the basis of diagnosis. They are encouraged to seek help solely on the basis of an unexplained deterioration in work performance. The decision to obtain the help is left to the individual employee, though failure to do so could result in termination if poor work performance were to continue.

Metropolitan Life

Metropolitan Life employs over 10,000 people at its headquarters. In 1941, a program was established to cope with behavioral disorders and alcoholism. In 1962, the Employee Advisory Service was created within the personnel department.

Confidential personal counseling is available for resolving personal and job-related problems. Five counselors serve about 4,000 clients annually. The problems handled relate to family strife, financial distress, alcoholism, substance abuse, job dissatisfaction, etc. Fifty percent of the problems relate to the family. Thirty percent of the problems arise from alcoholism. Eleven percent of the problems arise from medical disorders. Seven percent of the problems arise from drug abuse. Annually, about 600 employees are in counseling regarding retirement.

Counselors are selected on their ability to establish rapport. They must also have knowledge about company programs, financial planning, and benefits. They work closely with the medical department, from which they obtain inservice training. The training is provided by consulting psychiatrists, psychologists, physicians, and social workers.

How successful is the program? Eighty-five percent of the problems referred to the service are resolved in-house. The service is used by top management as well as supervisors and new employees. The program succeeds because employees have confidence and trust in its integrity. The director is in the field 23 days a year arranging for similar services in Metropolitan Life offices across the country (Egdahl & Walsh, 1980).

United Airlines

United Airlines offers an employee assistance program (Deneen & Hessellund, 1981). It is operated out of the corporate office in Chicago and is headed by a clinical director. The clinical director supervises five counselors scattered across the country. Three are located in California, one in Chicago, and one in New York. The counselors provide assessment, diagnosis, and referral as needed. They serve as rehabilitation case managers but also encounter such problems as employee stress, job difficulties, family dysfunction, addiction to drugs and alcohol, and need for legal and financial assistance.

Carvel Taylor, the clinical director, holds an M.A. from the University of Chicago in Clinical Social Work. She and the counselors are certified as alcohol counselors. The combined specialties of the staff include social work, rehabilitation counseling, psychology, and psychiatry. All have come to the program with previous experience.

Both salaried and timecard employees have used these services. Referral is voluntary, though supervisors are given instructions in confrontation techniques having to do with poor work performance. Since the program is housed in the medical department, referrals for physician care are easy to accomplish when necessary (Deneen & Hessellund, 1981).

Union Carbide's Nuclear Division

Union Carbide's Nuclear Division at Oakridge, Tennessee, operates a career-planning resource center. Information is maintained not only about the company but about careers generally (Trammel, 1980).

Out of the worker population of 11,000, 695 have volunteered to participate in a career-planning program offered by the center. Three services are offered:

1. A 50-hour self-evaluation workshop is given over seven weeks. An examination of the structure of the organization and of one's own goals are dealt with in the process.
2. Individual consultation is available. These sessions deal with employee's needs related to the world of work. Clients are helped to see how they fit into the structure of the organization.
3. Employees are instructed regarding the appropriate use of the career-planning center, including the library.

Reactions to this program have been favorable. Attendees say they have a better understanding of personal motivations, an increased sense of responsibility for their own careers, and a clarification of career objectives. Tests include an increased measure of self-confidence and a renewed interest in one's current job. Improvements have also been reported in the ability to communicate with supervisors. A greater awareness of the need to communicate accurately has also been discerned (Trammel, 1980). It is easy to see how the skills of the vocational counselor are used within this organization.

NASA Space Center

Supervisors at NASA's Goddard Space Flight Center participate in an elaborate career-development program (Leibowitz, 1980). By the spring of 1980, over 300 (out of 800) supervisors completed the course. A variety of activities are sponsored, including:

1. A performance appraisal system based on Civil Service Reform Act requirements which establish criteria for employee development.
2. A training program to help supervisors identify the strengths and resources of their employees and to use them productively.
3. Individual training plans to help employees obtain the experience needed to achieve their personal goals.

In the process, the center offers

1. Individual counseling by appointment only.
2. Instructions on how an individual may use the career-planning center by themselves.
3. An opportunity to summarize the results of their explorations.

IBM's Program for Career and Life Planning

IBM operates a program for career guidance and life planning (Marlowe, 1981). They call this program "Passages." It is conducted in workshop format and deals with actual life and work situations. The entire workshop requires 32 hours to complete, over 3 and a half days. A half-day follow-up occurs every two months. Its goal is to help employees answer for themselves the following questions: 1) Where have I been? 2) Where am I today? 3) Where do I want to go? 4) How do I get there? And, finally, as follow-up, 5) What have I learned?

The program was begun at the first manager level since these individuals have the greatest opportunity to advance in the company and are in a position to counsel the newest employees. The program content is designed to help the employee generate data about himself or herself and use this information as a means of formulating and implementing an individualized plan of action and to provide a follow-up opportunity for employees to evaluate their own progress. Structured evaluation questionnaires and appropriate standardized surveys and psychological tests are applied to achieve these goals. The overall learning experience is carried out with the assistance of work groups. Officials talk about goals of the company in the 1980s in order that the individual learning experience can be better applied to the actual work situation. Exercises are used to organize the data that has been obtained about one's own person and about the company generally. Individual counseling is available for developing individualized action plans. Homework is assigned so that individual plans can be shared with one's family. Follow-up sessions occur every two months in which progress on individual plans can be shared with the group and assistance by the group can be offered.

Ninety-four percent of those who have participated in the development of this program believe that the program should continue. There is a sense that it "is a nice thing for the company to do."

The IBM administrative staff concludes that career and life planning deserve emphasis in business and industry for the following five reasons. Such a program

1. Indicates to adult employees that the organization recognizes them as individuals;
2. Helps the individual prepare for changes in society, in the organization, and in themselves;
3. Effectively releases the potential of the individual in behalf of the organization;
4. Assists the manager and employee in jointly planning self-development opportunities;
5. Serves as a vehicle to improve communication between the manager and his or her employees. (Marlowe, 1981)

Career Guidance

In the preceding discussions, career guidance services were described as well as rehabilitation services. Career guidance is becoming increasingly important in human resources management. Columbia University surveyed 250 of the large Fortune 500 companies in 1979 (Campbell & Cellini, 1980). The following career planning services were offered to one degree or another within the surveyed group:

Career counseling with performance appraisal
Job rotation for career development
Individual self-analysis and planning workshops
Life- and/or career-planning workshops
Workshops on disengagement for retirement
Training supervisors in career development
Dual career ladder workshops

Utilization of "assessment centers"
Realistic job preview for new employees
Mid-career workshops
Dual careers for spouses

The obvious relationship between rehabilitation counseling and career guidance will, no doubt, continue to develop.

Conclusion

Industrial rehabilitation as a tool for managing people is not only used to restore the disabled to employment but also to maintain the self-confidence and psychological well-being of an organization's entire work force. The concept of managing people as a human resource involves more than the traditional personnel functions of recruitment, training, advancement, termination, and benefits administration. It involves a realization of "the good life" as a personal requirement on the job, and it takes into account both the beneficial and dysfunctional characteristics of the business in regard to the employee's well-being. The rehabilitation practitioner as a coordinator and counselor has always needed to understand the whole client and his or her fullest level of productivity. Human resources management assumes that all employees, disabled or not, are individuals and will have to cope with a variety of problems successfully so that their job performance will not suffer. The personnel function is broadening its concern to encompass a holistic approach to each employee. Rehabilitation techniques offer tools that can effectively be employed in this effort in the everyday management structure of an organization.

Traditionally, rehabilitation has been used to habilitate or to reinstate disabled individuals into the work force. Traditionally, counseling has been used in secondary schools and in colleges for guiding young people into careers. Today the fact that an individual may have several careers during a lifetime necessitates the transfer of these services to the adult population on a regular and ongoing basis. Industry, where automation, cultural differences, and changes in the economy affect the requirements of jobs, is beginning to understand that people must be accepted as they are and be assisted to be productive in an ever-changing work setting. Additionally, expectations of treatment for injury or illness necessitate effective rehabilitation of chronically ill and disabled people if a cap is to be placed on the ever-rising cost of employee benefits, particularly in respect to hospitalization, LTD, and workers' compensation. This is not paternalism. Paternalism only covers up the problem and hides the costs. Modern human resources management focuses on individuals' responsibility for their own performance with the requirement that they solve those problems which interface with effective work performance. Availability of rehabilitation services to augment health care, access to employee assistance programs through which an acceptable degree of homeostasis can be reached, and encouragement to utilize accessible career guidance services, all encourage a mutual responsibility between employers and workers.

The profession of industrial rehabilitation is on a frontier. The growing area of human resources management requires the maintenance of integrity, the capacity to market services, and the willingness to be flexible in using those services in a health maintenance capacity. As industry becomes enlightened to the benefits that accrue from an effective rehabilitation service, competent practitioners will be in demand.

References

Anderson, K. Personal communication, 1980.

Applebaum, S. H. Identification of factors and symptoms. *Health Care Management Review*, 1980.

Applebaum, S. H., & Davis, S. A. Man and organizations. *Industrial Management Review*, 1980, 69–79.

Campbell, R., & Cellini, J. Adult career development, *Counseling and Human Development*, 1980, *12*(10), 13.

Compshare brochure. 301 South State Street, Ann Arbor, Mich.: n.d.

Deneen, L., & Hessellund, T. *Rehabilitation of injured workers*. San Francisco: Rehabilitation Publications, 1981.

Egdahl, R. H., & Walsh, D. C. *Mental wellness programs for employees*. New York: Springer-Verlag, 1980.

Hoeffel, J. Personal communication, 1979.

Leibowitz, A. C. Career development center at NASA's goddard space flight center. *Career Development Review*, 1980.

Marlowe, A. F. Passages—A program for career and life planning. *Vocational Guidance Quarterly*. 1981, *29*(4), 355–361.

Martin, G. Fringe around the paycheck, employee benefits. *Occupational Outlook Quarterly*, 1980.

Rose, J. H. *Description of service*. Washington, D.C.: Joseph H. Rose and Associates, n.d.

Trammel, C. Career planning in Union Carbide's nuclear division. *Career Planning and Adult Development Newsletter*, 1980, *2*(12).

Welch, G. Testimony on behalf of Senate Bill 402, National Workmans' Compensation Standards Act of 1979. *Congressional Record*, March 28, 1979.

6 Organizational Consulting for Rehabilitationists

Thomas E. Backer

> Consultation is the providing of expert advice or guidance about how to best achieve certain individual or organizational goals to persons responsible for achieving them.
>
> —Backer, 1982

> A consultant is someone who borrows your watch to tell you what time it is. —Anonymous

These two contrasting definitions should help to give rehabilitationists an idea both of what consulting work is and some of the attitudes (good and bad) surrounding it. Learning the techniques of consulting and the professional attitudes that go with them are part of what anyone in the rehabilitation field must do in order to respond effectively to consulting opportunities in this area—helping an insurance company develop a monitoring system for its vendors, helping a federally funded rehabilitation research and training center get private rehabilitation firms to use improved practices springing from a research study, working with a manufacturing company interested in reducing its number of industrial injury cases, etc.

As far back as 1971, John Muthard compiled a catalog of rehabilitation consultants, which by its considerable length showed evidence of the number of professionals working in this capacity. The number has doubtlessly increased since then, especially the number of rehabilitation consultants making some (or all) of their livings in private practice (as opposed to those who consult as a staff member of a state rehabilitation agency or other public organization—often without fee). Service organizations in the private sector also may offer consulting services, either independently or as part of a larger operation (e.g., a progressive, high technology company offering both

Preparation of this chapter was supported in part by funding from the National Institute of Mental Health, Grant #32145.

management information systems for rehabilitation firms and technical assistance consultation in making such systems work smoothly).

This chapter has two main purposes. The first is to present basic concepts of consultation and a larger context of consulting practice to set them in, in order to clarify *process* issues in the private practice of consulting in rehabilitation. This material would be much the same regardless of whether one is a rehabilitation consultant or some other type of consultant. Second, the chapter will examine *content* issues, which are to some extent unique for rehabilitation professionals involved in consulting work, including the particular context in which consultation occurs (both professionally and societally) and issues relevant to training, ethical considerations, practice development, and the like. This chapter will focus on organizational consultation, though much of what is said also would be relevant to rehabilitationists performing individual case consultations, e.g., in a hospital setting.

Main topics the chapter covers are as follows:

- Types of consulting roles in private sector rehabilitation
- Distinctive features of consulting in rehabilitation
- The larger context: consultation in the 1980s
- Consultation and change: a basic concept
- Consulting roles for rehabilitationists
- Main activity stages in consultation
- Strategies for effective consulting: preparation
- Strategies for effective consulting: intervention
- Strategies for effective consulting: evaluation and follow-up
- Strategies for effective consulting: durability maintenance
- Training of consultants
- Practice development
- Fee setting
- Facilities and materials
- Developing a consulting organization
- Professional ethics
- Stresses and strains of consulting work.

The amount of theory presented here will not be especially great. Consultation is an activity of "doers" rather than "thinkers," so the literature on the subject is fairly small; most of what does exist is at the level of practice—case studies, intervention strategies, etc. In addition, virtually everyone holding a professional or managerial role in today's society does some work that could accurately be described as consultation. This includes a large number of people who would not define themselves as being consultants, and their work proceeds much more from practical experience than from any theoretical base.

Types of Consulting Roles in Private Sector Rehabilitation

As already mentioned, consulting on various issues of rehabilitation practice and the operation of rehabilitation organizations is nothing new, as John Muthard's 1971 directory establishes. Our focus here is restricted to rehabilitationists working in the private sector, i.e., persons who are at least partly in private practice and offer their professional services for a fee. These professionals may or may not also be associated with a larger organization, such as a private sector rehabilitation firm. Roles such consultants may take on include the following:

- Consulting to public sector agencies (e.g., on the development or carry through of rehabilitation research designs, on training of rehabilitation professionals, etc.); Backer (1981b) discusses consulting to the federally sponsored rehabilitation research and training centers and similar organizations.
- Consulting to private sector rehabilitation firms (e.g., on the development of services, on evaluation of services, on general administration, and on planning—all from the perspective of someone who knows the rehabilitation field well).
- Consulting to workers' compensation boards or other regulatory agencies, either as an expert witness or on larger organizational issues in legal determination, service delivery, etc.
- Consulting to insurance companies and self-insured private business organizations regarding selection of vendors to provide rehabilitation services, development of in-house rehabilitation programs, and so forth.
- Consulting to organizations about job safety programs for their employees to prevent or reduce industrial injuries and about organizational conditions that may facilitate or inhibit return to work of an injured employee. Lewin, Ramseur, and Sink (1979) discuss the work of rehabilitationists in industrial consultation from several of the perspectives mentioned above.
- Consulting to individual disabled persons and to organizations of persons with disabilities (e.g., individual case consultation in regard to litigation or consultation to advocacy organizations concerned with influencing public policy or legislation regarding the disabled).

There are, of course, consultants in the areas mentioned above who do not come from a rehabilitation background; for example, a private sector rehabilitation firm may well hire a management consultant rather than a rehabilitation professional to develop a personnel program. The rehabilitation consultant does bring special knowledge—especially about the complicated matter of rehabilitating persons with disabilities—to each consulting assignment. In many instances, the quality of input provided on such issues as personnel development, long-range planning, and the like will be enhanced by this background.

It should also be noted that the full-time consulting practice specializing in rehabilitation still represents a developing field—indeed, organizational consultation of all sorts is just now becoming reasonably well organized as a field of professional practice. Those desiring consulting work often may need to create valid opportunities to be of service to potential clients through their own background research and ingenuity. The opportunities are by no means limited to the ones just presented.

Distinctive Features of Consulting in Rehabilitation

Following are some aspects of consulting intervention in rehabilitation that are somewhat peculiar to this field:

- Rehabilitation has its own jargon, and consultants must be sure that they and their clients understand terms in relatively the same way (especially if the client is a private business organization).
- Rehabilitation often follows a medical tradition, with all the ramifications thereof (e.g., the unchallenged authority of the physician), especially when activities take place in a medical setting.
- Attention to issues of client advocacy and consumer involvement is important throughout the rehabilitation field today, including consultation.
- Rehabilitation is results-oriented more significantly than other human services—the "case closure status 26" model has a real impact on the way people think about programs and their results (including work initiated by consultants).
- Many rehabilitation organizations are public, nonprofit agencies—different than those in the private sector, including the way they seek out, use, and respond to organizational consultants.
- Many private sector rehabilitation firms, on the other hand, are inexperienced in using consultants, often because their principals are rehabilitation service professionals who have only recently become "business people," and may need some education before they can make full use of what a consultant has to offer.
- Rehabilitation involves a number of professional disciplines, often in a team atmosphere.

These factors should be kept in mind when reviewing the approaches to consulting presented later on in this chapter.

The Larger Context: Consultation in the 1980s

Accurate statistics about the many types of consulting activity going on in the U.S. are difficult to come by (Backer, 1981a). One estimate is that more than 2,800 firms and about 30,000 individuals (thousands of them independent, others members of a company or group) offer consultation to American public and private organizations (Fuchs, 1975). Another, from the May 21, 1979, issue of *Business Week* reports that "ACME . . . and *Consultants News* estimate the present number of consultants at anywhere from 25 to 50 thousand . . . easily three times what it was in the mid-1960s" (p. 99).

Organizational consultants include those who do consulting work on a part-time basis (often faculty members of colleges and universities), people in full-time individual practice, those in group practice of some sort on a small level, and finally members of fairly large to very large management consulting organizations. Typically organizational consultants are people trained in some content area such as business administration, engineering, or psychology, or anyone in dozens of other fields who have found a market for the knowledge, skill, and experience they have to offer. The *Business Week* article cited above quotes Joseph J. Brady of the Association of Consulting Management Engineers as asserting that "consulting is booming because the world is getting more complex." Increasingly, academicians are consulting on a part-time basis, and in a growing number of instances, they are converting to full-time consulting services, differing from the traditional model of "generalist" management consulting firms such as McKinsey & Company.

Types of Clients

All manner of individuals and organizations receive consultation. According to one survey (Shay, 1974), more than three-fourths of the nation's larger businesses and a host of smaller ones have utilized the services of management consultants. In addition, a number of federal, state, county and municipal governments, not-for-profit institutions, schools, colleges, universities, health organizations, associations, and foundations regularly obtain this kind of professional help.

Knowledge Base on Consultation

The overall literature on consultation is not a large one, but it is growing—as recent bibliographies by Mannino, MacLennan, and Shore (1975), Grady,

Gibson, and Trickett (1981), and Backer and Glaser (1984) point out. Some information resources for consultants will be presented in an appendix to this chapter.

Education for Consultants

There are no degrees in consultation per se as an identified professional field, and training programs in rehabilitation to the writer's knowledge pay no attention directly to this subject. Consultation is something people typically learn about through their own on-the-job experience, perhaps supplemented by a few readings or a single seminar. Issues involved in the training and education of consultants will be covered later.

Expanding Opportunities

Because consultants are marginal to the larger systems in which they operate and because they are problem-responsive (typically engaged to respond to specific difficulties or challenges experienced by an individual or organization), consultants tend also to be on the "cutting edge" of new developments. For example, human relations consultants were among the first to do work in what has become the "human potential" movement; popular topics such as stress management were first introduced widely by consultants to organizations. Consultants have played a substantial part in efforts now spreading all over the world to humanize organizations and, as a by-product, to increase productivity (French & Bell, 1973; for a specific example of an organization development program involving a consulting psychologist, see Backer & Seymour, 1980). Consultants have also helped to apply understanding of human behavior to creative work and the communications/entertainment media, such as the author's own work on stress management for actors (Backer, 1980), and psychological analysis of the creative process of film music composition (Backer & Manson, 1978). Rehabilitationists can project similar "cutting edge" opportunities for their consulting work—e.g., rehabilitation engineering, quality of worklife concepts as applied to rehabilitation service organizations, computers in rehabilitation, etc.

Consultation and Change: A Basic Concept

All consultation is oriented toward change consideration—helping individuals or organizations decide whether certain changes may promote goal attainment and if so, helping to implement the changes. Therefore, consulting work in rehabilitation involves helping people and systems to deal with the psychological ramifications of change—fear, resistance, for example, as well as with issues of technology, rehabilitation practice, legislation, community attitudes, and others.

While all consulting interventions start with considering the need for change, the end result may be either making the change or deciding quite deliberately not to make it—and perhaps even to reinforce the status quo. Consultants would do well to remember George Bernard Shaw's maxim, "If it is not necessary to change, it is necessary not to change." Change needs to be directed toward some concrete prediction of improved functioning, not just faddism or "change for change's sake."

Collaboration in planning change by all those who will be affected by it is clearly desirable in most cases. There can be great differences in the extent of collaborative planning associated with a change effort, however. For example, in the case of a badly needed change program—where working through staff resistances to effect meaningful participation simply may not be possible, given time constraints or other cogent reasons—change by administrative fiat ("do it or you're fired") may be the only viable solution. A consultant who recognizes such a reality may be able to influence the organization in that necessary direction more effectively than anyone on the inside.

Consulting Roles for Rehabilitationists

There are at least four distinct types of roles relevant to consulting work in the rehabilitation field:

1. A *problem-oriented expert* in some specialized field of knowledge or practice is one who comes in to diagnose and to help remediate or to perform a technical service in connection with some problem that the client feels unqualified (or hasn't the time) to handle independently or on which the client just wants another opinion before deciding on a course of action. A highly knowledgeable expert on workers' compensation laws in a given state, for example, might advise a company on how best to set up a corporate system that meets legal requirements.
2. An *advisor* helps sharpen issues, identify discrepancies, and perhaps shares his/her own relevant knowledge and experience. Here, the consultant does more than provide technical knowledge but generally does not work to develop an overall course of action. A consultant helping a worker safety program might be an example of this type.
3. A *technical assistance consultant* is called in by an organization

that (a) wishes to adopt or has adopted a new program or product and needs help to insure skillful implementation, at least in the beginning, or (b) has the need for revitalizing or stabilizing a current successful program. Here, the focus is on the specific problem about which the consultant has special knowledge, with the consultant making an effort to teach the client organization's staff how to solve the problem themselves. For instance, a consultant may help a rehabilitation facility plan for and install a computerized management information system.

4. *A process consultant* serves to facilitate basic organizational processes of planning, organizing, staffing, coordinating, motivating, and controlling, through which the organization can better define its own problems, conceive and implement its own solutions, and assess progress toward improved organizational performance. In the literature, this kind of consultant is often referred to as an "organizational development" (OD) consultant. The main emphasis is not on some specific problem but rather on the more general improvement of organizational functioning. A consultant who helps a private sector rehabilitation firm improve staff morale and communication through team meetings and counseling with the firm's top management is an example of work at the process level.

Main Activity Stages in Consultation

There are four main activity stages in consulting work:

- preparation
- intervention
- evaluation and follow-up
- durability maintenance.

The nature and intensity of each of these stages varies, of course, according to the type of consulting being done (expert consulting, for example, is mostly intervention with relatively little of the other three stages).

Preparation includes initial contact with the client to learn what intervention may be needed and set-up of a consulting arrangement or contract. Later aspects of preparation include doing whatever homework may be needed to prepare either for carrying out the initial diagnosis or revising it later on.

Intervention includes several steps: more detailed diagnosis of the problem or situation requiring action, prescription of certain activities that may be helpful in alleviating discomfort or making needed changes, engaging the client's involvement in that intervention process to whatever extent seems desirable given the circumstances, and then taking the necessary actions.

Evaluation and follow-up includes both informal and formal examination of what happened as a result of the consulting intervention and then taking whatever steps may be necessary to use what is learned to keep the intervention healthy as it moves along.

The last stage, durability maintenance, includes termination of the formal consulting intervention itself and planning for ongoing involvement as required to keep going whatever productive changes the consultant may have helped bring about.

The approach to conceptualizing consulting given here is a distillation of a variety of theoretical approaches to consultation. As Blake and Mouton (1978) have put it, conceptualizing or model building about consultation has typically involved a host of "warring camps"—theoretical positions derived close to the level of actual consulting activity by consultants working with one particular approach (e.g., private industry management consulting). Each of the warring camps has its own biases, and in other cases there may be biases about what the emphasis in the consulting process should be on. The statement here about theory has been deliberately brief in part to avoid getting into these areas of dispute.

Strategies for Effective Consulting: Preparation

Considerable evidence is now accumulating, both from a comprehensive interview study of 17 outstanding consultants to organizations (Backer & Glaser, 1979) and from the work of Judith Larsen and her colleagues at the American Institutes for Research (Larsen, Norris, & Kroll, 1976), to suggest that preparing for consultation is a critically important step that strongly influences potential for productive outcome of a consulting intervention. Perhaps even more important, Larsen and her associates have determined that both client and consultant need to get ready for consultation, and that some systematic preparation by both increases the potential effectiveness of consulting.

Naturally, the amount and degree of preparation that is most desirable depends upon the consultant's style and amount of experience, the nature of the consulting intervention itself, and the client organization. Highly skilled and experienced consultants may need to do relatively little in the way of systematic preparation; in psychological terms, they have "overlearned" the skills needed to perform their jobs. In other cases, the client organization itself and the consultation requested may set real limits on the amount of preparation that may be feasible or necessary. If the requirement for consultation is an urgent one, systematic preparation may be possible only to a very limited extent; the preparation phase may have to be cut short if the client's funds are tight and only a limited amount of support is available for the consultant's work. Also, some organizations may see extensive preparation as an unnecessary frill and might resist it to the extent that the consulting relationship could be damaged if the consultant continues demanding preparation.

The main steps in preparing for consultation are initial contact, preliminary problem statement, initial consulting arrangement, homework, and conceptual foresight planning.

Initial Contact. What happens as a result of the first telephone call or meeting with the client may set an enduring style for (and perhaps determine the effectiveness of) the interaction between client and consultant. The consultant may want to prepare a fairly standard list of questions about the client organization and the consulting request to help guide smoothly this first contact with clients.

Preliminary Problem Statement. Another set of questions may be used to elicit some initial understanding of what the problem or felt need is that led to the consulting request being made. Frequently, as in psychotherapy, a critical question is "Why now?" Organizations, like individuals, have problems, challenges, and unmet needs all the time—many are handled internally, left unresolved, or solve themselves by the passage of time. Why did the client feel the need to reach out for help at this particular point in time?

Also, what kinds of experiences has the client had with consultants before? What were the results? In particular, has the problem a consultant has been tapped to help with been addressed by a previous consultant?

Initial Consulting Arrangement. Once the consultant has determined that the stated problem is one he/she feels able to tackle, and there is evidence that the client has "learning readiness" with respect to taking action on the problem, the next step is to develop a preliminary understanding about what both consultant and client will be doing. In some cases, the client may require a written proposal laying out the work to be done and the cost of the consultant's doing it; in other instances, a simple letter of agreement may suffice.

Except for the briefest and most routine consulting interventions, having some form of written agreement between consultant and client is essential. How to write a full-fledged consulting project proposal is a broad subject beyond the scope of this chapter; elements in a basic letter of agreement include the following:

- *Who* is doing the consulting? (If you have colleagues or assistants who will be doing part of the work, this must be said to avoid unpleasant surprises later on.)
- *Who* is the client (in what parts of the organization will the consulting be done, and to whom is the consultant directly responsible)?
- *What* is to be done and in what time frame, and *who* in the client organization will be involved?
- What will be the fee and expenses and payment schedule?
- *What* is the client responsible for in terms of providing support, access to information, access to staff, etc.?
- *What* will be the mechanism for indicating that the consultation is complete, e.g., the delivery of a consulting report?

How to set fee levels is covered in another section of this chapter.

Homework. It generally is valuable for the consultant to review whatever written materials may be available which relate to the consulting work. This may involve nothing more than reading over a letter or two and an organizational brochure or annual report, and then jotting down a list of five or six items or questions with which the consultation may begin. Or it may be a much more comprehensive process, involving some hours of work in becoming acquainted with the client organization, or on occasion even designing a detailed intervention strategy prior to beginning the consulting work.

Conceptual Foresight Planning. The end result of preintervention planning is not a set of action steps cast in concrete! No good consultant goes in with a preordained approach to be imposed on the client whether it fits or not. While in some instances of expert, problem-oriented consultation, the advance definition of what needs to be done may be very precise and shared exactly by client and consultant, most consulting interventions involve a degree of ambiguity that is built into the reasons why the client has requested an intervention in the first place. Unresolved problems, uncertainties, and perhaps tensions or conflicts exist, but if the client could spell them out precisely in advance, outside consultation would probably be unnecessary. In fact, experienced consultants observe that the reason they are told they are being asked in to consult often turns out not to be the real or complete motivation for retaining their services.

Conceptual foresight — anticipating what events could happen during the course of the consulting intervention and planning for how the consultant will respond to each of these — is critical to success. For example, if the consultant has a clue that resistance may arise from a particular division or administrator in a client organization, how will that be handled? If it indeed turns out that a tentative hunch about hidden agendas proves true, what difference will that make in the subsequent actions the consultant takes? For highly experienced consultants, of course, a wealth of similar prior experiences tends to make their conceptual foresight machinery operate very quickly, often on an almost unconscious level.

An example may help at this point to specify how client and consultant can work together in getting ready for consultation. The author has consulted for several years with a large eastern public facility which provides comprehensive rehabilitation services. The consultation has typically consisted of one-day sessions whenever the consultant is in the client organization's geographical locality, usually about twice a year. Consultation has focused on a particular program within the organization, about which the consultant happens to have considerable prior background and expertise.

Each consulting intervention, although brief, is approached with considerable attention to planning and preparing. Once the invitation to spend a day in consultation has been made by the client, the first step is taken by the client organization in specifying (usually in the form of a letter) the topics to be addressed during the consulting intervention. These topics take the form of program areas where general input is desired or specific problems on which the consultant's help will be requested. Next, the consultant telephones the client organization's program director, and the list of topics is discussed. Reports and other materials pertaining to given topics of consultation are forwarded to the consultant for advance review (homework).

The next step is the critical one at the consultant's end. With materials and agenda of subjects to be covered in hand, the consultant typically spends most of the five-hour plane ride to the client organization's locality reviewing all available written materials and making notes regarding possible responses he may give to each of the identified topic areas. Typically, four or five pages of handwritten notes are taken—identifying questions to ask, specific resources to suggest, proposed intervention strategies for consideration by the client, and so forth.

In turn, the client organization's program director circulates the memo or agenda of topics to be covered by the consultant to program staff, and each person then prepares his or her own subagenda for group meetings.

Such planning activities have seemed to result in consultation visits that are extremely productive and that accomplish a great deal in a very limited amount of time. The evident reason for that productivity is good advance planning, thus minimizing the time required for "getting up to steam" or for the consultant to think of suggested approaches to dealing with the various topics of problems raised.

Strategies for Effective Consulting: Intervention

Main steps in the active intervention phase of a consultation are diagnosis, the prescription: goal setting and intervention planning, client involvement, and action.

Diagnosis. At this stage, diagnosis involves more than the previously mentioned "learning what the problem is about." Specifically, one is looking for information that will help to build the intervention itself, including needed data about the client organization. The consultant's sources may include written reports, staff of the organization (in which case all statements made should be cross-checked for accuracy!), and sometimes knowledgeable outside observers as well.

Probably the most influential exponent of organizational diagnosis as a consultation intervention technique is Harry Levinson, whose 1972 book centers on this subject. Levinson believes that the consultant must become immersed in the organization in order to diagnose its problems effectively. He has developed a comprehensive diagnostic outline based on his own consultation practice and on his years of teaching at Harvard. Since Levinson's approach to understanding organizational dynamics is based on principles of psychoanalysis, he tends to look for possible evidences of family relationships being played out in the work setting, conflicts of a Freudian nature, and so forth. However, psychoanalytic interpretations are not necessary to make use of Levinson's basic approach.

The types of data Levinson looks for in his organizational diagnoses include (1) basic identifying data such as what kinds of products or services the organization turns out; (2) historical data on the organization's development and growth; (3) how things are laid out physically throughout the organization and its various branches, if any; (4) the characteristics of employees (tenure, skills, absenteeism, turn-over rates, etc.), (5) how the organization formally goes about dealing with its people (recruitment, compensation, performance analysis, etc.); (6) what happens seasonally and with what urgency; and (7) how the organization gets data. Finally, Levinson would want to know what other experience with consultants the organization has had and with what results.

In many instances, the key to the consultant's diagnostic efforts will be looking at the organization, the consultation request and staff persons involved directly or indirectly in the consultation process, in order to determine what are the forces promoting or inhibiting change in the particular area the consultant has been asked to work in. A useful checklist for this purpose is one developed by Howard Davis of the National Institute of Mental Health, and summarized in the acronym A VICTORY (Davis & Salasin, 1975):

A. *Ability*: Resources and capabilities of the organization (staff training, facilities, funds) necessary to implement, sustain, and evaluate the change.

V. *Values*: Degree of accord between the values and attitudes required by the proposed change and the organization staff's existing attitudes, values, philosophy, and operating style.

I. *Idea-Information*: Clear communication to all concerned regarding the proposed innovation, evidence for its validity, and the techniques and action steps needed for implementation.

C. *Circumstances*: Relevant factors in the organizational environment that may affect successful implementation, especially those active at start-up time.

T. *Timing*: Timeliness of innovation attempt in regard to environmental factors.

O. *Obligation*: Perceived need for the innovation, and willingness of relevant decision-makers to authorize adoption.

R. *Resistance*: Inhibiting factors; organizational or individual disinclination to make the change for whatever reasons.

Y. *Yield*: Anticipated benefits or rewards from the innovation, as perceived by potential adopters and by those who would be involved with implementation at the operating level.

Once the consultant understands the kind of change program he/she is being asked to help implement and also has some initial understanding of the client organization, the A VICTORY factors can be reviewed either mentally or in discussion with the client. If there are serious deficiencies in one or more of these factors (e.g., the timing is bad for a new program, or staff resistance to it is predicted to be very high), there are three options: forge ahead anyway (but forewarned!), try to improve conditions before proceeding, or abandon the change program altogether. (Readers interested in more information about A VICTORY may consult Davis & Salasin, 1975, 1978).

Prescription: Goal Setting and Intervention Planning. This next step also varies greatly according to the situation, the nature of the client's request, the amount of resources available for consultation, and so forth. Setting specific goals for the intervention and engaging in systematic planning with the client participating in that process usually are critical to successful consultation.

Goal setting and intervention planning may constitute only a brief conversation with the client regarding what the consultant proposes to do, followed by the client's ready agreement and the consultant beginning work. Or it may entail a full-scale written proposal submitted for formal review by one or more key administrators or a board of directors. If clearly defined goals for the intervention are set at the beginning, both client and consultant will be more likely to know whether success has been reached at the end. Goals stated in a letter of agreement need to be reviewed in a face-to-face meeting between the consultant and all members of the client organization who will be involved in the consulting intervention.

Client Involvement. This critical, and often ignored, step actually begins with diagnosis—the client needs to be involved in both gathering diagnostic information and deciding what to do about it. Again, the degree of client involvement varies according to the situation and the style preferences of the consultant: some technically oriented expert consultants, for example, require virtually nothing in the way of involvement; the consultant simply offers expert input that the client accepts, modifies or rejects without any need for collaboration.

However, in most situations where significant organizational changes may be the by-product of the consultant's ongoing work, involvement both of key decision-makers and all organization staff who will have to live with the results of the change program is extremely important to success. Through this involvement process, resistances can be surfaced and questions asked. As a result, the consultant can receive valuable input from those involved at various levels with the potential change about how to do it, what side effects to expect, and so forth.

It is especially important that the consultant check with those who live in the organization about possible side effects of a proposed change program. For example, what effect may an intervention in one area of an organization have on other divisions or programs?

Action. Most of the specific action strategies a consultant might consider using in working with an organization will depend to some extent on the particular nature of the organization and on the nature of the issue on which consultation has been requested. Some general guidelines for action follow, adapted from Norris (1978):

1. *The consultant is goal-directed.* He or she exhibits this by such behaviors as
   - clarifying the frame of reference for the consultation;
   - clarifying the objectives and topics of the consultation;
   - maintaining the focus of the consultation.
2. *Activities are directed toward problem solution.* The consultant
   - helps to clarify the problem;
   - generates a number of solutions or action alternatives;
   - discusses the pros and cons of the proposed solutions;
   - discusses steps to implement possible solutions.
3. *The consultant encourages consultee participation.* He or she encourages participation by
   - asking consultees to establish priorities about what the consultation is to cover;
   - asking consultees to offer or generate ideas and solutions to the problem;

- asking consultees to come to consensus about workable ideas and solutions;
- listening actively and reflectively to consultees' contributions.

4. *The consultant is active rather than passive.* In addition to behaviors included in other categories, this means the consultant
   - is well prepared for the consultation;
   - provides examples, information, and references to other resources;
   - encourages consultees to anticipate the outcomes of implementing a proposed solution;
   - summarizes in terms of desired outcomes;
   - discusses ways to evaluate outcomes.
5. *The consultant keeps in mind the particular situation* when identifying, clarifying, and dealing with the issues of concern.
6. *In addition, the consultant*
   - highlights strengths;
   - is generally encouraging and supportive;
   - focuses on main concerns (rather than promoting his or her own agenda);
   - is effective in communicating information.

Strategies for Effective Consulting: Evaluation and Follow-Up

Traditionally, many rehabilitation professionals have thought of consultation as much like psychotherapy—consulting is clinical work, almost an "art form," and thus not readily subject to systematic evaluation. However, in recent years this philosophy has been changing, and there is now more professional pressure, and indeed more pressure from clients themselves, to evaluate consulting interventions with varying degrees of systemization (see Lippitt, 1981; Flaherty, 1979).

At the simplest level, evaluation may consist of nothing more than the consultant's returning to the client organization at some later date and asking whether the intervention was a success. Such requests for feedback will be a great deal more helpful if the consultant asks for specific examples of how the client knows whether or not the intervention was successful. These critical case examples can be valuable learning tools for the future.

Simple survey forms or questionnaires can also be used to obtain evidence of success. Particularly when the consultant has been working in an organizational setting to change attitudes or to increase knowledge about particular subjects, the success of consultation may be determined rather effectively by making written inquiries — of participants in training or team-building events, for example.

The highest level of evaluation involves conducting actual research on the impact a consulting intervention has had in an organization. Well-trained rehabilitation professionals such as psychologists may be especially qualified to carry out this kind of assessment because of their background in research methodology, statistical analysis, and so forth. At the same time, it is necessary to be realistic most consulting clients are not interested enough in formal evaluations to sponsor costs of such evaluations.

In designing any evaluation effort, questions such as the following need to be asked:

- What were the goals of the consultation, and by what specific actions or products can it be determined that these goals were achieved?
- What specific evidence of success or failure is actually available?
- How can this evidence be measured?
- What were the specific actions the consultant understood; who else was involved in the consultation and what did they do?
- How satisfied was the client with the consultation?
- How satisfied was the consultant with the consultation?
- How will the results of the evaluation process be reported?
- How will the results be used? (Such as a "report card" on the consultant, to improve later consulting efforts, etc.)

Strategies for Effective Consulting: Durability Maintenance

There is considerable evidence (e.g., Glaser & Backer's 1980 report on long-lasting innovations in mental health organizations) that not all worthwhile innovations, including those initiated by consultants, last over time. Frequently, and often because of deficiencies in the initial implementation stage, worthwhile programs flourish for awhile but then die out despite evidence of effectiveness and continuing need for whatever they provide.

All consultants to organizations thus need to be aware of the durability issues and recognize that initial success does not necessarily mean permanent success of an innovation or improvement they have helped in some way to bring about. Early planning for durability helps considerably. It is too late to begin durability-building efforts when the innovation is already flagging or in danger of being discontinued.

Helping the client organization, and especially key decision-makers in it, to understand the importance of planning for long-lasting success of an innovative program is also extremely important. Moreover, any change program or innovation (whether in procedure or technology) a consultant suggests should first be appraised in terms of what its likelihood for long-term success is in this particular organization, at this particular time (see earlier discussion on A VICTORY factors).

In conjunction with the above, the organization itself should be evaluated in terms of its likelihood of providing a continuing climate for success of the innovation. The point to remember here is that a change program that deteriorates or dies prematurely does no one any good; if a consultant learns that an organization is not likely to sustain a change effort over time, the most helpful intervention the consultant may then be able to make is to persuade the organization not to undertake the change program at all. A key factor for promoting durability is continuing involvement by the consultant, who may be in the best position to detect signs of lagging potential for durability.

Training of Consultants

Typically, a rehabilitation professional starts consulting both with the background of formal education and full-time employment in a particular area, e.g., a counselor's position in a state rehabilitation agency or a faculty post at a university. To move from that beginning into consulting work requires careful self-definition, acquisition of knowledge, and professional skill development.

Content knowledge can be sharpened through readings and course work: the consultant needs to make a particular effort to keep abreast of what is new in his or her chosen specialty field; clients expect and have a right to "the latest" when they buy a consultant's services—not the mindless implementation of fads but the thoughtful evaluation of recent developments for adoption or rejection as governed by the client's particular situation. Continuing education programs offered through NRA, NARPPS, or other professional organizations may also be helpful in this regard.

Most rehabilitationists starting out as consultants also will need training and preparation regarding the process of organizational consultation itself. As already mentioned, technical expertise is not enough; consultants also need to understand the dynamics of organizational change, the psychology of individuals within an organization that is changing, and the communication processes that are necessary to develop and carry through worthwhile change programs. These "process sides" of the consultant's professional skills are rarely attended to in degree programs or in the direct work experience of most human service professionals. Readings, seminars, and special workshops or training programs offered at universities or elsewhere are among the ways one can acquire such skills.

In addition to specific skills relevant to making consulting interventions, some more generic characteristics a consultant needs to possess are to some extent amenable to training. Perhaps the most important is a problem-solving style—an action orientation to move into the client system and provide tangible help. Although philosophies about intervention may differ, all consultants need to help clients understand and decide whether change may be desirable. To do so requires an ability to help the client perceive the pros and cons of various change options, along with a willingness to become involved enough with the client to understand the organization and the particular problem(s) on which consulting input is desired. Also, a growth orientation, as a part of professional development and continuing education, appears to be essential for consultants, especially those working in large organizations where there are so many challenges associated with intervention in widely different, complicated environments.

The most frequently mentioned approach to teaching people how to be consultants (according to the Glaser and Backer study of outstanding consultants to organizations) is apprenticeship. Apprenticeship involves the opportunity to work with an experienced consultant in order to learn both the specific skills of consultation and a general philosophical/professional orientation. For example, a beginning consultant in the insurance industry might go along with a trained colleague on an assignment with a large insurance firm, mostly observing what takes place during the interaction and perhaps making more specific input in a subject area in which the "beginner" is already an expert.

Apprenticeship has the key advantage of offering real-time experience in organizational consultation. However, two other approaches to training consultants that need to be considered (particularly because the supply of "masters" to the number of "apprentices" seeking training may prohibit everyone using this approach) are training through readings on consultation and training courses on consultation offered by various universities and private organizations.

Some selected readings are given in the appendix to this chapter. At present, the best access to the literature in this field is provided by *Consultation*, a national-circulation magazine about organizational consulting also described in the appendix. In evaluating the potential utility of any consultation training course, the first step is to decide what kind of consulting one wants to do and with what clients (or what sort of practice has already been developed by a given individual). Then, the cost and time investment of the training course can be weighed against its potential for helping to develop needed skills and a professional orientation. The professional societies listed in the appendix, plus one's colleagues in the consulting field, are the best sources of information about training programs that might be of value.

Practice Development

As already suggested, the consultant's first client often comes along "by accident"; a referral by a colleague, a former student, or some other source that the newly defined consultant did not actively seek out starts the ball rolling. To continue consulting work, however, some marketing of one's services is necessary so as to make potential clients aware of one's availability and then to persuade them to offer an engagement (this subject is covered more extensively in Backer & Glaser, 1981). Useful techniques for practice development include using brochures, advertising, referrals, public service events, professional appearances and publications, serendipitous marketing, general media and print appearances, booths at conventions, and public relations consultation.

Brochure. An attractively formatted, easy-to-read prospectus of the services one offers as a consultant is a marketing tool that can be used in many ways. For example, the brochure serves to remind prospective clients what services the consultant offers and can be used to share that information with others in the prospective client organization besides the particular individual with whom one has had an initial contact. Sometimes mailing of a brochure with a suitable cover letter to an identified group of potential clients can be helpful, though the percentage of response will not likely be very great.

Advertising. Until very recently, many human service professionals were more or less forbidden by the code of ethics of their professional group to engage in any significant amount of advertising activity with respect to professional services. Now, however, there have been some changes, and although any consultant establishing an advertising policy would do well to consult the relevant ethical standards before taking action, it is safe to say that at least a certain amount of low-key advertising now is permissible, and an increasing number of consultants are in fact engaging in advertising.

Referrals. The two most important sources of referrals are one's professional colleagues (even other consultants, especially those in different geographical areas or whose type of practice is different from one's own) and present or past clients.

Public Service Events. An increasingly popular approach to obtaining business is offering informational lectures or seminars to groups of people likely to include prospective clients.

Professional Appearances and Publications. Giving papers or participating in symposia at NRA, NARPPS, or other professional society meetings may spur referrals. Colleagues who hear the consultant at these events become aware of the areas of expertise she/he has to offer, and often consultants can insert appropriate references to their work as consultants. Publications in the professional journals (including those possibly read by one's potential clients) on topics one is competent to write about—and therefore presumably competent to consult about—also can be of value.

Serendipitous Marketing. Referrals often are made through the channel of social interaction, appearances at charitable or educational functions, and so forth. Particularly for those with a highly unusual service to market—one that may be requested almost as soon as a prospective client becomes aware of its availability—these contacts can be extremely important.

General Media and Print Appearances. Some consultants, especially those who operate at a high level (e.g., the chief executive) in large organizational settings or who offer consultation in interesting or unusual subject areas that would be appealing to the general public, find that marketing appearances on radio or television shows and preparing articles about subjects related to one's consulting services for popular publications are useful marketing approaches.

Booths at Conventions. Events like the Abilities Unlimited Expo in Los Angeles, which draws together many private and public sector organizations in the rehabilitation field, can provide excellent business development opportunities. In addition to taking a booth, brochures and other printed materials may be distributed during such convention appearances.

Public Relations Consultation. Only very recently has it become even marginally acceptable for professionals to have public relations consultation in developing their reputation, general visibility, and image. Now, however, an increasing number of professionals in all areas, from medicine to psychology to law, are retaining public relations consultants on a part-time basis to help them engage in all of the above activities.

A major alternative for full-time consultants is to seek a position with an already existing organization such as a private vendor. This often can be a permanent organizational home; or, in other cases, several years of employment in such an organization may develop enough contacts and expertise about the consulting process that it may then be possible for the consultant to go out on his or her own or even to start an independent organization. Naturally, a consultant considering such a move must be certain both that he/she is qualified to practice independently and that the move is made with proper regard for professional ethics.

The practice development techniques described here are hardly the only ones a consultant may use to develop a successful consultation practice. In some cases, one may derive as much consulting work as is desired through a single client, e.g., a former employer. Rehiring retired employees as consultants is common practice both for private employers and government agencies.

To many traditionally trained rehabilitation professionals, at least some of the above marketing and business development approaches may seem undesirable, commercial, or extreme. However, it is clear that more commercially based marketing approaches for consultants are here to stay. It is obviously an individual decision how much one takes advantage of such techniques. But the professional values and ethical codes are changing, and practices unacceptable 10 years ago (such as advertising) are acceptable today. The alternatives presented here are hardly to be endorsed for all professionals in all circumstances; however, many might be given serious consideration as part of the approach by which a rehabilitationist can work to develop an ethical, responsible, and successful consulting practice.

Fee Setting

The consultant's clear definition of service area or professional specialty can help in the fee-setting process, which is often difficult at best. Particularly since many professionals until very recently have been prohibited from advertising or even openly discussing fees, it has often been difficult to get an idea of what it is reasonable to charge. There is now more widespread knowledge about fees, but much still depends on the area of consultation and the geographical setting in which the client organization resides, as well as on such obvious factors as the consultant's reputation and degree of expertise.

Often, the best place to start in the fee-setting procedure is to ask a colleague who currently offers consultation in the same general area about fee structures. Input about comparable fees also may be sought from CPAs, attorneys, and other types of professionals in one's geographical area. Generating some rules of thumb to guide fee practices may also be helpful, such as the common one of offering a somewhat lower consulting fee to public or third sector organizations as opposed to those private business clients one has.

Facilities and Materials

Since many consultation practices start out of the consultant's home, or from the office of an existing full-time job, beginning a practice may involve no more than obtaining occasional secretarial services for the typing of reports.

As a practice expands, however, the requirements often become much the same as for any other kind of business: an office, suitable office equipment, business cards and stationery, telephone service, secretarial services, and other customary business support services as the consultant's practice grows. Many consultants also find it useful to develop certain kinds of routine backup materials to be used with clients.

The consultant also needs to decide which professional or trade associations he or she wishes to join in regard to consulting work. Some may choose to restrict their professional associations to those in the rehabilitation area such as NRA plus regional or state associations; others may decide to join organizations that offer specialty benefits to consultants, even if that means associating with a large number of people who are not from the rehabilitation field. Local or national trade associations that bear upon the content area of one's work also can be possibilities. The appendix to this chapter mentions some professional associations for consultants that may be considered.

Developing a Consulting Organization

There are four types of consulting firms an individual may wish to start:

- *A partnership of full-time consultants.* The partners may employ additional associates if needed, generally with opportunity for the employees to advance into partnership after some years of satisfactory association.
- *An association of individuals who share certain overhead costs*, such as rent and secretarial services, and where one may cover the practice of another during vacations or illness, but where each associate fundamentally is in practice for himself and derives his income from his own billing minus his share of overhead costs.
- *A sole proprietorship or a corporation*, insofar as legal form is concerned, with mainly part-time associates who carry out certain types of consulting activity only through and "under the banner of" the firm with which they are associated.
- *A sole proprietorship or a corporation*, insofar as legal form is concerned, with mainly full-time staff employees.

Naturally, the decision as to which type of organization best suits a particular consultant depends heavily on the individual's goals—whether one prefers to work independently or as part of a group, one's profit orientation, and so forth. And many consultants may never wish to grow beyond independent, solo practices.

Professional Ethics

Guidelines for professional conduct of consultation, of course, begin with the ethical standards typically of a professional background in the human services. Principles specifically relevant to consultation include

- The client must be informed of risks or costs associated with the consulting intervention.
- Client organization staff (not just top decision-makers) need to participate in the consulting work as much as is feasible, especially in setting goals.
- Some sort of evaluation of the consulting intervention's impact is important.
- The consultant needs to be very careful about potential conflicts of interest, either between the needs of the client organization and his/her own needs or desires, or with any of the consultant's other clients.
- The consultant must be careful to stay within his/her area of expertise in providing consulting services.

More specific ethical pitfalls in consultation work have been identified in interviews with outstanding consultants to organizations (Backer & Glaser, 1979):

- Misuse—for the consultant's own personal gain or power needs—of close relationships that may develop with authority figures in the organizations.
- Failure to recognize that the consultant is serving the organization in a resource capacity, not running it.
- Violation of confidences or of confidential information that may be acquired in one way or another and failure to inform client of the limits of confidentiality.
- Invasion of privacy, sometimes coupled with failure to protect against possible misuse of reports the consultant may generate regarding individuals' personal characteristics.
- Failure to avoid conflict of interest or actively seeking significant favors from clients.
- Temptation to prolong a consulting engagement beyond what is needed, useful, or productive, chiefly in order to continue billing. The consultant should avoid alternatives which strengthen dependence of the client on consultant in favor of alternatives which strengthen the client's own internal resources or which call upon ap-

propriate resources outside the organization, for example, other consultants with special sets of skills.

- Failure to give each individual or group with whom he/she consults, regardless of organizational status, the very best one can offer in terms of respectful attention and concern.
- Failure to realize that in some situations the process of helping management improve its lot may be at the expense of the organization or workers at large. The ethical issue is to be aware of this possibility at the front end, then to decide whether one wishes to proceed — or whether management can be helped to seek an essentially "all-win" modus operandi.
- Failure to recognize one's own limitations of competence and to avoid making exaggerated claims or failure to recognize when one is no longer effective, especially when finding that the modus operandi and/or the goals of the client are incompatible with one's values.
- Failure to speak out to the client if an action is perceived as wrong, destructive, or counterproductive, despite contract arrangements that have been made.
- Failure to think through with the client possible negative side effects of a given consulting intervention or proposed approach to a problem and to consider whether the potential gain is worth the foreseeable risks.
- Failure to plan with the client for necessary follow-through on interventions before undertaking them; e.g., if an employee opinion and perception survey seems warranted, is there a plan and commitment for follow-through into timely problem solving, with employee participation in that process?
- Failure to assess organizational readiness for given changes and to keep "readiness" criteria in mind during the implementation stage.
- Failure to present realistically the results of a program or intervention.
- Failure to maintain objectivity and independence and the need to avoid seduction into being used by one part of an organization — such as by a boss to invade a subordinate or a rival's privacy or serve as an organizational "spy" or as a "hatchet man."
- Temptation to impose one's own values, such as for complete openness and frankness, on people who do not feel comfortable with such behavioral styles.
- Failure to be nonjudgmental and respectful toward other consultants and disciplines.
- Resistance by the consultant to evaluation of his/her own consulting efforts.

Using one's own observations and input from the client can help to avoid these pitfalls.

Stresses and Strains of Consulting Work

Consulting is a demanding occupation: it requires a high level of expertise, entails for most independent or small-group-based consultants a considerable level of risk in a strict business sense, involves many hassles of travel and scheduling, and demands a high level of energy and commitment. Consultation can also be an exciting and rewarding activity, which may more than offset the psychological or physical stresses and strains it involves. The effective consultant is one who recognizes that the stresses and strains are real, anticipates them, and takes steps to deal with the problems that result.

Probably the key to managing stresses and strains effectively (in consultation or any other kind of human activity) is conceptual foresight—the ability to anticipate what problems may arise from a given course of action and then to devise in advance solutions or partial solutions that may help to deal with these problems if they occur. For example, a consultant may anticipate what resistances can be expected to emerge in a client organization as a result of proposing certain alternative courses of action. Then the consultant can schedule time to deal with these resistances rather than having to either ignore them or needlessly sacrifice personal energy and convenience to deal with them when they arise unexpectedly.

A second important technique for handling these stresses and strains is processing; that is, periodically reviewing one's consulting work to identify where problems are recurring so changes may be made in one's consulting style to reduce or avoid these. For example, certain kinds of consulting assignments may almost inevitably entail the strain of too much or too sudden travel requirements. The consultant may decide as a result simply not to accept engagements of this sort; without stopping to look at one's professional work as a consultant on a periodic basis, however, these operating problems may be obscured. Over time, a consultant may do much to adjust the way in which his or her practice is operated so as to reflect personal priorities and needed areas of growth for the consulting practice or organization as a whole. Again, processing can help to make these decisions.

Finally, a simple philosophy: one should not expect work as a consultant to be easy! Gearing expectations to certain difficulties and stresses and strains simply makes it easier to tolerate the problems when they do occur while continuing to enjoy the considerable rewards and satisfactions being a rehabilitation consultant can provide.

Appendix: Resources for Rehabilitation Consultants

This appendix has three sections: (1) a listing of books and journals about consultation; (2) descriptions of professional associations for consultants that rehabilitationists might be interested in; and (3) a description of the Consultation Research Program, an NIMH-funded project conducting many activities relevant to consultants in the rehabilitation field.

Print Materials

The following are some brief annotations of publications that would be of interest to consultants in the rehabilitation field.

Backer, T. E. *Principles of technical assistance consultation for rehabilitation personnel.* Washington, D.C.: George Washington University Rehabilitation Research and Training Center, 1981.

A booklet describing briefly some essential principles of consultation in the rehabilitation field, focusing on consulting assistance to public rehabilitation organizations in the research and training areas.

Glaser, E. M., Abelson, H. H., & Garrison, K. N. *Putting knowledge to use: Facilitating the diffusion of knowledge and the implementation of planned change.* San Francisco: Jossey-Bass, 1983 (developed under support of the National Institute of Mental Heath).

An extensive literature review, including summaries of hundreds of works on organizational change.

Goodstein, L. D. *Consulting with human service systems.* Reading, Mass.: Addison-Wesley, 1978.

A brief text designed mainly for those who wish to consult to human service agencies.

Lippitt, G. L. Evaluating consultation services. *Consultation*, 1981, *1*(1), 17–26.

An excellent theoretical and practical discussion of evaluation issues for the consultant, which focuses on concepts organized under Lippitt's model of the evaluation process.

Lippitt, G. L., & Lippitt, R. *The consulting process in action.* La Jolla, Calif.: University Associates, Inc., 1978.

An excellent "primer" text on organizational consulting—brief and well written and offering a variety of case examples from the authors' own consulting experiences.

Professional Societies

Some organizations that rehabilitation consultants might wish to join include the following:

Academy of Management, Division of Managerial Consultation
Terry L. Maris
Eastern Illinois University
Charleston, Ill. 61920

The Academy's membership consists largely of business school professors and is oriented toward management research; the Division of Management Consultation is a special interest group again largely of academic orientation. Membership requirements are based primarily on interest in activities of the division.

Division of Consulting Psychology (Division 13), American Psychological Association
Mack T. Henderson, Membership Chairperson
Rohrer, Hibler & Replogle
626 Wilshire Boulevard
Los Angeles, Calif. 90017

A group of almost 1,000 psychologists whose professional practice includes provision of consulting services to organizations. Requirements for membership include the Ph.D. in psychology and professional interest in consultation.

Institute of Management Consultants
19 West 44th Street
New York, NY 10036

A certifying body for individual management consultants, granting the designation C.M.C. (Certified Management Consultant). Membership restricted to individuals who spend more than half of their time consulting, and an examination is required.

International Consultants Foundation
5605 Lamar Road
Washington, D.C. 20016

Registry of consultants doing international consulting, designed to stimulate cross-cultural consultation work.

Society of Professional Management Consultants
41 East 42nd Street
New York, NY 10017

Individuals and consulting firms are both represented in this group, which has high membership standards and is oriented especially toward general management consultants in the private sector. Members reflect a broad spectrum of services in a wide variety of disciplines and industries serving business, government and associations.

Consultation Research Program

A six-year grant (1979–1985) was awarded to the Human Interaction Research Institute in Los Angeles by the National Institute of Mental Health to establish and operate this program, directed by Dr. Thomas E. Backer and Dr. Edward M. Glaser. CRP has conducted research, training, product development, and dissemination activities. Many of its products (more than 150 in all have been issued since 1979) will continue to be available at cost after the close of the project, including the most comprehensive bibliography on organizational consultation now in existence.

Consultation, the magazine for organizational consultants published as part of CRP's dissemination and utilization activities, will be published commercially after the end of 1984. For information on subscriptions to *Consultation* and other publications mentioned above, contact: Mr. Dann Grant, Project Coordinator, Consultation Research Program, Human Interaction Research Institute, 10889 Wilshire Boulevard, Suite 1120, Los Angeles, Calif. 90024 (213) 870 1373.

References

Backer, T. E. Coping with stress. *Screen Actor Newsletter*. December 1980, 4–5.

Backer, T. E. Organizational consultation: Where we stand in 1981. *Consultation*, 1981, *1*(1), 5–11. (a)

Backer, T. E. *Principles of technical assistance consultation for rehabilitation personnel*. Washington, D.C.: The George Washington University Medical Center Rehabilitation Research and Training Center, 1981. (b)

Backer, T. S. Psychological Consultation. In J. R. McNamara & A. G. Barclay (Eds.), *Critical issues, developments and trends in professional psychology*. New York: Praeger, 1982.

Backer, T. E., & Glaser, E. M. *Portraits of 17 outstanding organizational consultants*. Los Angeles: Human Interaction Research Institute, 1979.

Backer, T. E., & Glaser, E. M. *Developing a professional practice as a consulting psychologist*. Los Angeles: Human Interaction Research Institute, Consultation Research Program, 1981.

Backer, T. E., & Glaser, E. M. *Bibliography on organizational consultation*. Los Angeles: Human Interaction Research Institute, Consultation Research Program, 1984.

Backer, T. E., & Manson, E. L. In the key of feeling. *Human Behavior*, 1978, 7, 63–67.

Backer, T. E., & Seymour, T. F. Personnel development in a small firm — A psychological viewpoint. *California Accountant*, 1980, *35*(5), 5–7, 10.

Blake, R. R., & Mouton, J. S. Toward a general theory of consultation. *The Personnel and Guidance Journal*, 1978, 56, 328–330.

Business Week. The new shape of management consulting. May 21, 1979, 97, 99–101, 104.

Davis, H. R., & Salasin, S. E. The utilization of evaluation. In E. Struening & M. Guttentag (Eds.), *Handbook of evaluation research* (Vol. 1). Beverly Hills, Calif.: Sage Publications, 1975.

Davis, H. R., & Salasin, S. E. Applied social research: In combat with waste and suffering. *International Journal of Comparative Sociology*, 1978, *19*(1–2), 107–113.

Flaherty, E. W. Evaluation of consultation. In J. J. Platt & R. J. Wicks (Eds.), *The psychological consultant*. New York: Grune & Stratton, 1979.

French, W. L., & Bell. C. H. Jr. *Organization development: Behavioral science in-*

terventions for organizational improvement. Englewood Cliffs, N.J.: Prentice-Hall, Inc., 1973.

Fuchs, J. H. *Management consultants in action*. New York: Hawthorn Books, 1975.

Glaser, E. M., & Backer, T. E. Durability of innovations: How Goal Attainment Scaling programs fare over time. *Community Mental Health Journal*, 1980, *16*(2), 130–143.

Goodstein, L. D. *Consulting with human service systems*. Reading, Mass.: Addison-Wesley Publishing Company, 1978.

Grady, M. A., Gibson, M. J. S., & Trickett, E. J. (Eds.), *Mental health consultation: Theory, practice, and research 1973–1978: An annotated reference guide*. Washington, D.C.: National Institute of Mental Health, Department of Health and Human Services, 1981.

Larsen, J. K., Norris, E. L., & Kroll, J. *Consultation and its outcome: Community mental health centers*. Palo Alto, Calif.: American Institutes for Research, 1976.

Levinson, H. *Organizational diagnosis*. Cambridge, Mass.: Harvard University Press, 1972.

Lewin, S. S., Ramseur, J. H., & Sink, J. M. The role of private rehabilitation: Founder, catalyst, competitor. *Journal of Rehabilitation*, 1979, *45*, 16–19.

Lippitt, G. L. Evaluating consultation services. *Consultation*, 1981, *1*(1), 17–26.

Mannino, F. V., MacLennan, B. W., & Shore, M. F. *The practice of mental health consultation*. Washington, D.C.: USGPO, 1975.

Muthard, J. E., & Crocker, L. M. *Directory of rehabilitation consultants*. Gainesville, Fla.: University of Florida, 1971.

Norris, E. L. *Getting the most from program-oriented mental health consultation*. Palo Alto, Calif.: American Institutes for Research, 1978.

Shay, P. W. *How to get the best results from management consultants*. New York: Association of Consulting Management Engineers, 1974.

7 Characteristics of the Private Rehabilitation Client: Implications for the Rehabilitation Specialist

Shelia S. Newman, Debra A. Perry, and Elizabeth L. Pan

Introduction

Very little published information exists about the private rehabilitation client — who he or she is in terms of age, educational background, marital status, or type of disability. This chapter attempts to pull together what is known about the private rehabilitation client, relying when necessary on unpublished data provided by private rehabilitation agencies, as well as the authors' own experiences. It is hoped that this chapter can increase the understanding of those who are serving the private rehabilitation client, not only in terms of dealing with his or her own frustrations on the job, but also in terms of advancing the state-of-the-art of private rehabilitation service delivery.

Private rehabilitation clients may include those injured in nonwork-related accidents and those disabled by long-term illness, but the majority of clients served by private rehabilitation agencies are injured workers who receive workers' compensation benefits. This subset of the population — the industrially injured — is the focus of this chapter.

In order to put this population into perspective, it is important to note that although the level of industrial injury and disease is high, the majority of such cases do not require physical or vocational rehabilitation. For example, of the 3,045,048 reports of occupational injury and disease recorded by the Liberty Mutual Insurance Company between 1971 and 1975, 87% of the workers returned to work before they were eligible for disability payments. Sawyer (1976) further reports that fewer than 2.5% of the total number of cases received benefits for 63 days or more. It is within this latter group that rehabilitation efforts may be required, and this is a very small percentage of the total population of affected workers.

On the surface, the rehabilitation of injured workers may appear to be a relatively simple process of vocational counseling. The client who has a work history might be expected to transfer skills easily from a previous job that is no longer physically possible to a new job that is within the physical limitations imposed by the disability. While work skills, prior work history, and developed work ethic are favorable to rehabilitation, the unemployment rates among industrially injured workers are far above what would be expected based on physical impairments alone (Conley, 1976; Conley & Noble, 1978). It appears, therefore, that there are additional issues that derive from the characteristics of the injured worker and the nature of his or her situation that are relevant to rehabilitation. The discussion of these issues constitutes the second purpose of this chapter.

The environment in which rehabilitation services are delivered also gives rise to issues that the rehabilitation specialist has to deal with. Discussion of service delivery issues and trends constitutes the third major objective of this chapter.

Who Is the Injured Worker?

Because private-sector rehabilitation is a relatively new field, comprehensive and nationwide statistics on caseload characteristics have not been adequately collected and disseminated. However, by examining data from several sources and combining these with the experiences of field workers, some conclusions about the client served by the private sector can be made. In this section the authors present available data on the demographic and other characteristics of the injured worker: occupational and educational background, type of injury, age, sex, and marital status.

Occupational Background and Status

One of the most important characteristics of the injured worker as a rehabilitation client is the existence of prior work history. This characteristic is generally considered as a favorable factor in determining the likelihood of placing the client in a competitive job. However, as the data below indicate, the predominant occupational background is blue collar—work that typically requires physical abilities. The loss of these abilities through injury can render the specific work history irrelevant in relation to the client's skills for another type of occupation. In many cases, the compensation received in the prior job cannot be matched by another occupation, a factor that contributes to the difficulty of placement.

International Rehabilitation Associates, Inc. (IRA) (1981) identifies occupational groups in which their clients can be categorized as follows:

% of Total	Occupational Group
65.4%	Labor-blue collar including construction and heavy assembly
13.3%	Office workers
9.0%	Professional employees
12.3%	Miscellaneous

The reader is cautioned that the above data include auto liability and long-term disability cases.

Another factor to be taken into consideration is the lapse of time between injury and the provision of rehabilitation services. Often the client has not been working for a few months, and more typically a year or more, before rehabilitation services are begun. Sanchez et al. (1981) report that almost a year elapses from injury to rehabilitation service in the state of California. This period of time is probably even greater in states where the laws are not as favorable toward rehabilitation and the system is not as well developed. Typically then, the injured worker who is referred for services in the private sector has been vocationally inactive for many months.

Educational Background

The lack of information on the educational background of the industrially injured worker is particularly acute. However, considering the fact that most injured workers are in blue-collar occupations, it can be logically deduced that the educational history does not include graduation from high school. This is in fact what Beals and Hickman (1972) found in their study of 180 industrially injured males from the state of Oregon. They noted the average length of schooling to be 8.96 years. The experiences of many private-sector rehabilitation specialists support the projection that typically the injured worker lacks a high-school diploma.

Type of Injury

Sampling case closures of workers in California who had been involved in rehabilitation in 1979, Sanchez et al. (1981) found the following statistics with regard to injury:

46% had back injuries
15% had knee injuries
12% had hand injuries

8% had neck injuries
4% had head injuries
4% had leg injuries
4% had wrist injuries
4% had elbow injuries
3% had shoulder injuries

The most recent figures available from IRA (1981) indicates that its national caseload has the following disability characteristics:

41.7% had lower back injuries
20.3% had fractures
10.4% had sprains and dislocations
6.2% had lacerations and contusions
3.3% had major multiple injuries
2.3% had amputations
1.7% had burns
1.5% had minor multiple injuries
1.4% had contusions
1.2% had crush injuries
10.0% miscellaneous disabilities

The IRA caseload includes clients who were referred under automobile liability and long-term disability coverage as well as workers' compensation. In both examples, however, back injuries are the most common type of injury encountered, with a variety of other orthopedic injuries also prominent.

In comparison, the 288,325 persons rehabilitated by state vocational rehabilitation agencies in 1979 had the following major disabling conditions:

21.0% orthopedic impairments caused by accidents, spinal-cord injury, cerebral palsy, and a variety of other disabling conditions
20.3% major disability or mental illness
12.1% mental retardation
9.2% blind or other visual impairments
6.2% deaf or other hearing impairments
5.1% digestive system conditions
4.7% alcoholism
3.0% genito-urinary system conditions
1.3% drug addiction

The remainder included a variety of disabling conditions such as epilepsy, heart disease, respiratory system conditions, etc. (U.S. Dept. of Education, 1979).

It would appear from these statistics that public rehabilitation programs serve a population with more severe disabilities than do private sector programs. However, it should be noted that the private sector data are incomplete, particularly with regard to secondary disabilities that may in fact be a primary obstacle to rehabilitation. Emotional illness, alcoholism, and drug addiction may be present and/or aggravated by the injury or may develop as a result of the injury.

The incidence of mental retardation has also not been tallied. Specialists report experience of having an injured worker psychologically and vocationally tested for placement or retraining and learning that the individual may be mentally retarded or of borderline intelligence. So, while the incidence of physical disabilities is known because it is the basis of the referral, little is known about the prevalence of other disabling conditions that could pose major barriers to rehabilitation efforts.

Age

Age is another factor relevant to rehabilitation efforts. The young are medically resilient and often more adaptable to change. Sanchez et al. (1981) report data based on case closures in California (see Table 7–1).

Table 7–1. Relationship of Age to Successful Rehabilitation

Age Range	*% of Total of All Injured Workers Medically Eligible for Rehabilitation*	*% of Total of All Injured Workers Successfully Completing Rehabilitation*
21–25	8	7
26–30	10	18
31–35	15	18
36–40	13	18
41–45	13	14
46–50	12	14
51–55	12	4
56–60	9	7
60	5	0

Mean age: 31½ years

Most of the workers medically eligible for rehabilitation fell between the ages of 31 and 50. These figures indicate that workers who drop out of rehabilitation are more likely to be under 26 and over 50.

Figures from IRA (1981) also indicate that many clients of this private sector company fall between the ages of 31 and 50. The 0- to 18-year-old category predominantly reflects other than workers' compensation referrals. Their age characteristics are as follows:

0–18	6.5%
19–30	28.3%
31–40	23.0%
41–50	19.8%
51–60	16.0%
61 & over	6.4%

(mean age = 37 years)

State agencies serve a larger group of under 18 year olds, which skews their figures. State agency age characteristics are as follows (U.S. Dept. of Education, 1979):

Age at referral	% of total caseload
0–18	11.8%
18–19	9.6%
20–24	17.0%
25–34	24.1%
35–44	15.3%
45–54	12.6%
55–64	7.0%
65 & over	2.5%

(mean age = 32.6 years)

Sex

State agency caseloads have a fairly equitable sex distribution: males comprise 53.3% of their caseload, and females 46.7%. IRA (1981) statistics indicate that 66.4% of their caseload are male. Lynch's (1979) review of several surveys of injured workers also lends support to the premise that the worker's compensation client is more likely to be male.

The predominance of male clients in the private sector caseload is not surprising since most injured workers represent blue-collar occupations such as construction, mining, and laboring positions — traditionally male-dominated occupations.

Marital Status

IRA's (1981) statistics indicate the following characteristics with regard to marital status: 66.5% are married, 22.6% are single, 6.8% are divorced, and 2.7% are widowed.

In contrast, state VR agencies report (U.S. Dept. of Education, 1979) that 31.6% are married, 44.0% are single, 12.7% are divorced, and 4.5% are widowed.

These figures indicate that the private sector client is more likely to have certain established roles within a family structure. Considering the fact that private sector clients come from the working classes and are middle-age males, these roles are more likely to be that of the traditional breadwinner. The effects on rehabilitation and the counseling implications of these factors will be considered later in this chapter.

Composite Profile

The picture that emerges from available data suggests that the injured worker is likely to be male, middle-aged, and married. He is typically a blue-collar worker who lacks college training and probably has not completed high school. His disability is likely to be the result of a back injury; however, the rehabilitation specialist can expect to deal with a range of physically disabling conditions. Typically, the worker will have been out of work for several months, or perhaps even several years. In some cases, hidden disabilities may be present. However, there is no documentation to support the incidence of substance abuse, mental retardation, emotional illness, and other disabilities since rehabilitation services are usually requested because of occupational injury.

This review of the data is not intended to create a stereotype of the private sector rehabilitation client. The authors' purpose is to highlight factors that will be further explored in this chapter because they are significant to the provision of vocational services to this population.

Psychological, Financial, and Related Issues

Although demographic data tell us something about the rehabilitation client in the private sector, they do not explain why one client is successfully returned to work while another, with similar characteristics, is not. In this section, we will explore psychological, financial, and other issues specific to the rehabilitation of the injured worker.

Reaction to Trauma

One of the first considerations in the rehabilitation of the injured worker is the effects of the traumatic event of injury. Although major effects of this trauma may have been diffused before the client is referred to the private rehabilitation specialist, this is not always the case.

Typically, people have similar reactions to trauma, or any stimuli which they are unable to master by flight, fright, or problem-solving behavior (Keister, 1971). This set of reactions, which Keister calls the traumatic syndrome, includes anxiety, startle reactions, insomnia, nightmares reliving the accident, sweating, palpitations, headaches, dizzy spells, blackouts, sensitivity to noise, and other signs of depression such as decreased sexual drive, irritability, withdrawal, and finally, regressed behavior leading to increased dependency. The individual's psychological equilibrium is disrupted by the trauma. His ego is weakened, and he may lose self-esteem. At a time when reassurance is needed, blame and conflict often result.

Asher and Asher (1976) point out that experts disagree whether this series of symptoms is simply a reaction to change or a form of mental illness. Keister (1971) estimates, however, that a large portion of the benefits paid to compensate physical symptoms are necessitated by traumatic neurosis.

The rehabilitation specialist must be aware of the complexity of psychological reactions to trauma. Although the specialist may not be involved in the early stages, he or she should be alert to the behaviors described. Protracted personality changes, unusual emotional reactions, and avoidance of the work task are other symptoms of traumatic neurosis that may be encountered (Asher & Asher, 1976). Whether or not the reader subscribes to the psychiatric label, such a behavioral response must be recognized since it could be a severe obstacle to rehabilitation.

Reactions to Changes in Lifestyles

When work is disrupted, the entire lifestyle is disrupted because the workers' lifestyles are often based on their jobs and the income they generate. Lynch (1979) notes that because the situation is sudden, the worker is often unable to deal with the physical, social, psychological, vocational, and financial implications of the injury. This is especially true when marriage and family structure are based on the worker's occupation.

An attorney who represents workers' compensation clients (Treon, 1979) states that the client misses the lifestyle that included the status and self-esteem that goes with working every day and performing a good day's work. He or she usually hates the "always underfoot at home" routine.

Whatever else the lifestyle included at the time of injury, it did include going to work every day, and that is no longer possible.

The role changes that result in the family can cause loss of self-esteem. A case from the Washington, D.C., area is typical:

> At forty-three, this client sustained a back injury that prevented him from continuing his work as a brick mason. He, his wife, and four children moved to the D.C. area six years before the accident to escape the South's slower economy. Following the accident, the family was very supportive, but as financial pressures mounted, so did family tension. His wife finally went to work when bill collectors could no longer be put off. Because of his wife's new work responsibilities, the client assumed the housekeeping responsibility for the entire family. "The kids won't listen to me, can't understand me, and won't respect me anymore," he complains. Neither he nor the family could understand why his back would not improve or why he could not lift, bend, or stand or walk for any period of time. Once the family provider and decision-maker, he has come to feel dependent and inadequate.

Peterson (1980) reviewed several studies and concluded that marital disharmony often results when role changes occur. This is especially true when the married partners adhere to the stereotypical husband and wife roles, as in the case of many workers' compensation clients who work in traditional construction, manufacturing, and mining industries. Many marriages end not only as a result of role changes but simply because the lifestyle that included houses, cars, and clothes that were afforded by credit are no longer available to the nonworker.

Loss and Mourning

The issue of loss is another factor that has particular relevance to the injured worker. Although the physical loss may not appear great as compared to other more severe or long-standing disabilities, the injured worker experiences many types of loss. This factor is therefore considered worthy of extensive consideration since loss of physical functioning, activity, social contacts, identity, lifestyle, and perhaps job are experienced by the injured worker who is referred for services. Consider the following case:

> Harry was 42 years old. He fell off a ladder while changing a lightbulb at work. He had been a diesel mechanic for over twenty years and worked for the same company for eight years. He planned to retire with them.
>
> The accident didn't seem too bad; Harry hurt his knee. Later he learned that he smashed it so badly that the knee cap had to be removed and that he severely damaged all the muscles. For a man past his prime, healing would be slow.

Harry missed the contact he had daily with everyone at the shop. His co-workers used to stop by after work, but after a year, their visits were few and far between. Financially, Harry was making it with his compensation benefits, but he missed those extra dollars he used to spend on weekend barbecues and parties.

Now that he's up and around a little more, he can make trips to the grocery store and drive himself to physical therapy. Luckily, his wife is still working. Two kids are at home. The oldest, a boy, is starting to work to pay part of his expenses.

Harry misses his old life. He's just recently realized that he won't be able to return to his old job. He's never been a desk or office worker, but it looks like that's where he is headed. He wonders how much he can earn in a new field at his age and is afraid about starting a new career.

Harry's case illustrates the loss that injured workers may experience in all realms of their lives: loss of physical functioning, loss of a body part, loss of friends and social contacts, loss of daily routine and activity, loss of identity (as a worker and a breadwinner), loss of established family role, loss of status, and loss of financial security.

The whole concept of stages of mourning as a reaction to loss were originally identified by Elizabeth Kübler-Ross as a result of her work with the terminally ill and their families. She identified the stages of mourning that begin with initial shock followed by denial, anger, resentment. A bargaining stage is common, followed by depression and sadness. Acceptance results if the individual passes through the other stages (Kübler-Ross, 1969). The stages of mourning have been applied to a variety of loss situations including loss of limb (Parkes, 1975), loss of job (Finley & Lee, 1981), and loss of physical functioning due to disability (Hughes, 1980).

This process can apply directly to the injured worker's situation. Hughes (1980) in his discussion of loss as it pertains to physical disability emphasizes that the grieving process is both a reaction to loss and a recovery process. It is evident that rehabilitation specialists must understand, accept, appreciate, and facilitate the grieving process if they are to successfully understand and deal with the behavior and feelings of their clients. The specialist who denies the impact of the physical disability or the loss caused by the injury, or who encourages the client to deny the implications, is actually preventing the client from facing up to the reality of the situation—and thus progressing.

For many injured workers, even the nature of their loss may be confused or unclear. Orthopedic injury and soft tissue damage may take many months and even years to reach a point of medical stability. Their medical outcome, security of their jobs, and the stability of their relationships may be tentative. Lack of clarity in relation to the loss could prolong the stages of mourning.

Kowalsky (1978), a rehabilitation nursing consultant, noted her frustration in trying to apply the Kübler-Ross stages to her patients. She found that individuals with disability do not pass through the stages in an orderly fashion; they may slip from one stage to another. The concept of "triggering experiences" was useful to her. Basically, the grieved individual may appear to reach a point of stability in relation to the disability, and then some event will cause upheaval and regression. It may even initiate the entire process again. These triggering experiences are usually events which are reminders of the loss, or in the case of disability, the limitations it imposes. Examples of triggering experiences are marriage, starting school, and job selection. Such situations require that the individual reconfront the loss experience and the limitations that result. This concept has obvious implications for the injured worker who may be about to embark on a retraining program or a return to work.

In summary, loss, like trauma, cannot be precisely calculated. The individual's experience is based on his values, identity, and the meaning of the disability incident to his life. Awareness of loss, and the possibility of loss in many areas of the injured worker's life, will help the specialist to understand what may appear to be negative and self-defeating behavioral patterns. The literature indicates that the mourning process is in fact a healing process. The specialist needs to assist the injured worker in passing through these stages so that they will be able to move along to the vital stage of accepting the loss and to continuing to build a productive life.

The Accident Process

Hirschfield and Behan (1966; Behan & Hirschfield, 1963) offer a different perspective to the loss and grieving process. After analyzing 300 cases of industrially injured patients, they concluded that these accident victims played an active role in the causation of the injury. They believe that the loss encountered as a result of injury serves the purpose of changing the socially unacceptable disabilities of the injured workers they studied into more socially acceptable ones. Their studies illustrate that the preexisting emotional status of their patients may be a critical factor in the causation of the injury and outcome of the rehabilitation process.

Simply stated, the dynamics of the accident process start with an event or situation that produces increased anxiety, tension, stress, or depression. The individual experiences difficulty coping with the situation and the feelings it elicits. Feelings of dependency become intense, but they are denied. The individual is unable or unwilling to seek help to alleviate the emotional conflict. As a result, competence and ability to function decline. This is an unacceptable disability to the individual. According to Behan and Hirschfield, injury is the solution (often unconsciously motivated) to this irresolveable conflict. After the accident, the inability to function, the distress, and the poor performance have an acceptable, uncontrollable, and external cause and is therefore considered acceptable.

The following case study from Hirschfield and Behan's original article illustrates the accident process:

> Consideration of these multiple meanings of work goes far toward explaining the injured man's conflict. If one pictures such a laborer who is required to lift a 25-lb. weight three times a minute for 8 hours a day, an easy example is established. Usually this work rate, agreed upon by both union and management, assumes the average worker's age to be about 28. If the worker in our present example is 52, he may come to the doctor saying that his 25-lb. weight is four times as heavy. X-rays show a normal lipping of the vertebrae for the patient's age. In plain language, this means that the man's back is quite different from that of a man whose age is approximately half the patient's. The worker in question is facing loss of his only salable commodity. At least unconsciously, he is losing the purpose and challenge of his life. He is also losing the main thing that he has to do, and most of his opportunity for social life is slipping away. On an inner level, he is losing his strength, his masculine identification. In addition, his economic basis of life is disappearing. This man's status quo heralds bankruptcy, so his depression is hardly a mysterious symptom.
>
> The conflict which this man must endure now becomes understandable. He wants his position, his masculinity, his social and economic life, but he also yearns to escape pain and the ever-increasing weight of the stock he has to lift every 20 seconds. His position is like that of a soldier on the battlefield, who wants to stay and be a man. The conflict and the anxiety resulting from it are acute. Both can be relieved with a partial solution—the soldier who is hurt does not have to fight, and the sick laborer doesn't have to work. (Hirschfield & Behan, 1966, pp. 115–116)

Hirschfield states that in post-injury the patient may avoid physicians who may in fact help alleviate the physical symptoms, thus unmasking the underlying unacceptable problems. Weinstein (1980) points out that the accident can result in increased self-esteem resulting from the acceptable disability. Secondary gain factors such as social and monetary reinforcements can further the disability syndrome and help explain the tenacity with which some disabilities are maintained.

It should be noted that the individuals whom Hirschfield and Behan studied were all involved in litigation and demonstrated emotional difficulties. The extent of physical and psychiatric damage resulting from the injury was being determined. The nature of this sample precludes generalization to all injured workers. Even so, the private rehabilitation practitioner will probably find value in considering the implications of the accident process as it relates to certain injured workers. It suggests that many psychological disturbances may not be a result of the injury or even have been aggravated by the injury. These difficulties may have in the first place triggered the accident.

Resistance to Counseling

It might be assumed that the mental and emotional aspects of disability would make the injured worker not only accept but seek counseling. Experienced rehabilitation specialists, however, indicate that this is not always true. One of the reasons offered is the fact that it is usually the client's first experience with counseling. Many people see counseling as asking for help and thus a sign of weakness. They are reluctant to admit that they cannot solve their problems alone. When these people are already receiving compensation, they may tend to view counseling as giving up yet another facet of their independence. Many injured workers say they come to counseling because the insurance carriers say they must. When the client is male, experienced specialists expect even more resistance to the counseling process.

Carlson (1981) suggests that men are more likely to try to cope alone and thus remain "unaffected" by problems that occur, such as their injuries. Counseling is seen as the expression of vulnerability, pain, and confusion, all of which should not be experienced by the stereotypical male. Scher (1981) states that men are often constrained by their roles and find change difficult. They are raised to believe that autonomy is the highest good. Therefore, the experience of being counseled is likely to create inner turmoil to the male who has prided himself as being able to make it alone. The rehabilitation specialist must be aware of this resistance and interpret it correctly. Involving the clients in all decisions and giving them responsibility will be likely to lessen resistance, in that they feel less "helped."

Responses to Conflicting Parties

Even without a rehabilitation specialist, injured workers are confused by the number of people involved with their attempt to return to work. These parties can include the employer; an insurance carrier representative; the employer's attorney; the client's attorney; rehabilitation nurses; physical therapists; occupational therapists; a maze of doctors, including orthopedists, neurologists, physiatrists, and psychiatrists; an administrative agency representative; a judge; a rehabilitation counselor from the state agency; union labor officials; the private rehabilitation specialist, and more.

In addition to the number of people involved, clients must also deal with conflicting information from the different parties. Therefore, injured workers often misunderstand their rights. They can only see that they have suffered an accident, a disability, and are undergoing complete disruption of lifestyle and career. They feel rejected by employers and pulled in different directions by their attorneys and doctors.

Lynch (1979) reports that injured workers often feel that insurance carriers are telling them one thing, attorneys another, and their employers yet another. In addition, injured workers often see a number of physicians, each giving a slightly different diagnosis and presenting a different treatment. The physiatrist may tell them they have weak trunk muscles, the psychiatrist may explain that situational problems are at the root of their difficulties, the neurosurgeon may describe a ruptured disc, and the orthopedist might find mechanical defects. All of these conflicting reports tend to confuse the injured worker and to promote a feeling of distrust toward the people who are supposedly there to help them.

> Lynn is a good example of a client who is confused by the number of people and the conflicting information she has received since her accident. Lynn worked as a cook until she slipped and injured her knee. She has had two surgeries and most likely always will walk with crutches. Soon after her injury, one doctor released her to return to light work while another advised her to have surgery. Her employer offered her light work. When she followed the advice of the second doctor and refused employment in order to schedule surgery, the insurance carrier cut her benefits. She hired an attorney, and her benefits were restored while she was in the hospital. She called the state vocational rehabilitation office to see if she were eligible for vocational counseling. She received a medical evaluation and was tested, but before she got too far, a rehabilitation nurse from the insurance carrier visited her and scheduled an appointment for a specialist from a private rehabilitation agency to see her at her home as soon as she returned from the hospital. She called her state counselor and her attorney, who both advised her to keep the appointment. In all, Lynn estimates that she has talked to or listened to about twenty people. She still doesn't know her legal rights and is afraid of counseling and the insurance company.

Fear can be further increased when clients talk to other injured workers who have experienced an adversary relationship with the former employer and the insurance carrier. When compensation checks cease, as in Lynn's case, clients who are not informed as to why or when the last check is coming can be expected to react negatively. This only creates further distrust that interferes with the return to work. Eaton (1979) outlines the difficulties the insurance carrier can create when representatives indicate that the company's financial losses are more important than the physical and medical problems of the injured worker. Indifference on the part of insurance carriers and tardiness in payments of compensatory benefits are barriers to rehabilitation. Smedley (1976) reinforces this point of view by pointing out that insurance carriers are not by nature rehabilitation-oriented. They are ial agents whose major responsibilities are to their policyholders or ,eholders.

The insurance carrier or former employer who does not understand the complexities of problems inherent in compensation cases may accuse injured workers who are not cooperating with rehabilitation of malingering. Sooner or later these clients will probably be forced to participate in legal proceedings while attorneys question the client's doctor and employer's doctor about whether or not the client can return to work. Asher and Asher (1976) describe the adversary atmosphere as being yet another factor that is detrimental to the rehabilitation of injured workers. Unless the client's attorneys are involved in the rehabilitation process, they, too, can hinder rehabilitation efforts. Not all clients are represented, but even when they are, they may express confusion about their rights.

Attorneys who question legitimate medical reports and instruct their clients to reject job offers do so most often in cases that are being resolved through court hearings (Eaton, 1979). No matter what the reason, the client who is instructed by an attorney to do one thing, an insurance company and rehabilitation specialist another, and a doctor yet another, becomes confused about his or her rights. Eaton indicates that the injured workers' misconceptions about their rights is a barrier to rehabilitation. Whether or not an attorney or counselor explains the rights, many injured workers believe they justly deserve monetary settlements. They do not understand the compensation laws and that lump-sum settlement or guaranteed payments are not automatic. Eaton suggests that they may attempt to improve the probability of a large settlement or the promise of continuing payments by prolonging their pain and the handicapping effects of the injury. Attorneys are often accused of encouraging this type of behavior when settlements are indicated.

Another problem that can add to the confusion and mistrust is that many laws deny a worker the free choice of a physician. Workers who do not trust the physicians chosen by the insurance carrier will often ignore the advice to seek rehabilitation and may sabotage rehabilitation efforts. In addition, doctors often don't understand the specific duties of many jobs. They write a "return to light work slip" when the industry cannot offer light work, and the injured worker is sent home. However, the insurance carrier who is informed of the return to work authorization will often cut benefits, causing further confusion and resentment on the part of the client.

Labor unions can further add to problems created by the other parties involved in the case. Not providing information is one problem. Clients are reluctant to explore work options without knowing what they may stand to lose. In many cases the loss can be great.

Conflicting information and the obstacles faced by dealing with so many people can leave injured workers confused and distrustful. Lynch (1979) suggests that the confusion and distrust can then lead to uncertainty, fear, and anxiety, which in turn decrease the injured workers' pain tolerance. The rehabilitation specialist can reduce these obstacles by coordinating services and efforts of the various parties. The specialist must be a negotiator, educator, and public relations person as well as a counselor. Each party should be involved in the return-to-work plans and be made to understand the impact the party's actions can have on the worker. Specialists must understand the compensation laws and learn to deal realistically with medical, social, and vocational issues.

Chronic Pain

Pain is a frequent factor observed in workers' compensation injuries, especially back injuries. Lynch (1979) reports that pain is the basic variable that is common to all low-back injured workers.

Bond (1970) notes that low-back problems result in more difficulties for both employees and employers than any other disability. Chook (1972) says that low-back pain is one of the most common yet difficult to manage chronic illnesses among industrial workers. Back injuries and resulting pain cost more than one billion dollars annually in disability funds and consume 20% of all compensation payments made in any given year, according to Fey and Fordyce (in press).

People who have low-back pain and back injuries are both those who do heavy physical labor and those who sit for the majority of the day. Magora (1972) found that people who are able to stand intermittently on their sedentary jobs have far fewer incidences of back problems. While back problems occur at about the same frequency in sedentary jobs as in heavy labor, the latter are most frequently referred to private rehabilitation agencies, for obvious reasons. The people who do not lose time from work are skilled workers or clerical workers already in light-duty positions. Their cases may only require job modifications, if any rehabilitation activities are indicated. It is the chronic cases that most often are referred to private rehabilitation. Sometimes these cases have been through litigation or are facing litigation, and they are referred as a last attempt to return the worker to gainful employment before the carrier cuts compensation payments or the injured worker faces court hearings. Samuel is a good example of this situation.

> Eight months ago, Samuel's doctor reported that he had recovered as much physical function as he could and that he should seek a different line of work. Because of his back injury, he could not return to his occupation as a truck mechanic. Rehabilitation was recommended.
>
> Samuel was referred to a private rehabilitation agency. He expresses a great deal of anger and resentment toward the former employer who insisted

that there was no light duty work available for him. He reports that he is unable to work full-time because of the pain he experiences. He has not explored any other occupations and is reluctant to consider anything that offers a lower salary than his former job.

Bond (1970) adds to this profile with his suggestion that workers similar to Samuel often show evidence of poor adjustment to life's circumstances —they have difficulty in coping with family and financial problems.

Fey and Fordyce (1983) believe that injured workers (or any person who has chronic pain) soon learn pain responses in order to put off making life decisions. They believe that pain sometimes serves to remove the person from a difficult or stressful situation and that temporary solutions are based on pain behaviors. Other writers, however, stress that the person who was once able to deal with problems is so inundated with pain and confusion that he or she now requires help to sort out the solutions to the problems. The whole person must be considered, and when the client is helped to break down one problem at a time, the chance for success becomes greater. The client in pain cannot focus on a return to work when other problems are increasing the amount of pain experienced.

The authors have worked with clients whose pain is reduced when outside problems are resolved. Often, if a significant problem, such as a large debt or a marital conflict, can be resolved the pain will subside enough to allow rehabilitation to start.

Employers find it difficult to understand back pain. Since it is difficult to determine how long soft tissue injuries take to heal, employers must often fill the vacant job before the injured worker is ready to assess whether he or she cannot return to that occupation. They often become resentful of the former employer and fearful of the future. The resulting anxiety can produce both more pain and a lower tolerance to it.

Injured workers often go from doctor to doctor, receiving different diagnoses. They usually become frustrated, angry, manipulative, and frequently noncompliant, according to Fey and Fordyce (1983). Narcotic habits that result from pain medications can eventually mask the original problems.

The case of Tom, while not intended to be representative of all back injuries, is a good example of some of the clients a rehabilitation specialist in a private agency can expect to see. It can be used to illustrate some of the complicated factors that result from back pain initiated by an on-the-job injury.

Tom has been off work for five years, receiving compensation benefits as a result of an accident during the construction of a sixteen-story building. Tom was an electrician and earned about $18,000 five years ago. The compensation he received is two-thirds his pay at the time of the injury. The law that governs Tom's claim does not allow for a cost-of-living increase for temporary payments such as Tom's. Tom was referred to a private agency three years ago but was not happy with the alternatives he saw for himself. When his doctors disagreed about the amount of physical activity he could resume, he tried to go back to his former job. He could not cope with the pain and exacerbated his injury level. Tom misses his former occupation and insists he would rather be earning the $25,000 his former co-workers now earn as construction electricians. He had surgery last year, but it did not increase his functioning ability or lessen the amount of pain he experiences.

During the five years of his disability, Tom had to sell his home and move outside the city to be able to afford to live on the compensation payments that do not allow for inflation. His wife has returned to work but has made it clear to Tom that she prefers to be at home. She admits that one of the things that first attracted her to Tom was the fact that he earned "a lot of money" and that he was strong and masculine. She now views him as being weak and unable to provide for the family. She does not understand why he can't return to work. She says he looks as strong as he ever did.

Tom realizes that he is close to a divorce. Even his relationship with his children has deteriorated. He used to be the one to discipline the children, but his wife has taken over that responsibility, too. He views himself as a failure as a role model for his three sons and one daughter. He seldom leaves the house as he insists he must lie down often to relieve his chronic back pain. He takes large doses of muscle relaxers and pain medication. He has become addicted to percodan, an often-prescribed pain medication. Tom's new counselor reviews all these circumstances with him and refers him to a pain program.

Tom is typical of the clients who report to pain programs. Fey and Fordyce (in press) describe the typical person who reports with a complex variety of problems built during long years of physical disablement: inactivity, high levels of pain behavior, narcotic addiction, depression, some forms of sexual dysfunction, and vocational difficulty. A brochure for an Ohio pain clinic states that the average pain clinic client has had back surgery and has sought in vain for pain relief for six to eight years.

In Tom's case, the doctor and counselor worked together to combat Tom's years of inactivity and his inability to face the reality of the disruption of his life and career. He was slowly relieved of his drug dependency, and he and his wife were referred to marriage counseling. Because he had to move to a rural area, his occupational options are limited but he has begun to explore the possibility of on-the-job training in a less physical field.

Reactions to Invisible Disabilities

Tom's case also illustrates the problems that an invisible disability can create. His wife finds it difficult to understand his limitations since there is no difference in appearance. Injured workers complain that their limitations are 'erlooked by professionals, peers, employers, and even family mem- omments such as "I wish I were in a wheelchair so people would at ecognize that I can't do all the things I used to do" are sometimes heard by rehabilitation specialists.

In addition to having the pain and "nothing to show for it," there are often no physical findings to support the complaints of pain and disability unless there is an obvious ruptured disc. This fact alone makes the compensable back injury a difficult case to manage and to understand. The specialist must be able to view the client holistically and help him or her separate personal, medical, and vocational problems and deal with all of them to ensure a return to gainful employment. Smoller and Schulman (1981) suggest that activity and involvement are critical. The client should be encouraged to share feelings, and the family should be involved in the rehabilitation process.

Secondary Gain Reinforcement

Malingering is an often applied explanation for the lack of progress in many workers compensation cases, especially back injuries. Malingerers are described as financially secure and comfortable about receiving compensation benefits. The malingerer supposedly makes conscious decisions to "play sick" and "rip off the system." Actually however, malingering is thought to be rare, according to Beals and Hickman (1972). Asher and Asher (1976) point out that while malingering is common shortly after most accidents, the temptation to malinger is overcome by guilt, shame, or honest values. A desire to return to the previous lifestyle is common.

In fact, numerous other issues and dynamics—social, psychological, and financial—can account for what appears to be active resistance to return to work. Collectively, these are called secondary gains of disability. Behaviors, circumstances, or events which reinforce the disability status or sick role are secondary gain issues. They serve to perpetrate symptoms. Unlike malingering, the process of seeking secondary gains is unconscious. Some authors have used the term "compensation neurosis" to label the process that involves maintaining symptoms and avoiding rehabilitation to maintain the financial and emotional security disability provides.

The inclination to seek out secondary gain reinforcement can result from the preinjury personality of the individual. If immature or dependent, the individual will be more susceptible to the reinforcing value of secondary gain circumstances. Ross (1971) points out that the results of trauma can reduce inner strength and coping, thus increasing the disposition toward secondary gain dependencies. Secondary gain gratifications can result from three types of need areas: dependency, retaliation, and avoidance. A disability may mask underlying dependency. Compensation benefits, sympathy, and increased attention can maintain fragile self-esteem. Dependency has an acceptable uncontrollable cause.

Secondary gain can also be in the form of retaliation against an organization or an individual, according to Ross (1971) and Asher and Asher (1976). The injured worker may feel gratified because his or her injury is costing a resented employer financial hardship. Unjust treatment by an employer can serve to perpetuate the disabling effect of the injury and lead to maximum benefits (Asher & Asher, 1976). This can be particularly true in cases of negligence. The desire to blame someone or to place responsibility on some party for the injury—the feeling that someone must pay for the suffering and injury endured—can also serve as an incentive to seek maximum benefits. Such retaliatory secondary gain can also be directed toward a spouse or other individual who is burdened by the injury.

Secondary gain can also be derived from the reinforcement gained through avoiding unpleasant, uncomfortable, or fear-inducing situations. Avoiding hard, demanding, or boring work, fear of failure, fear of a career change, or the fear of confronting one's own difficulty in handling one's life situation prior to injury are just a few examples.

The fields of medicine rehabilitation and psychiatry recognize the implications of secondary gain for the rehabilitation process. Secondary gain reinforces the sick role and encourages the maintenance of symptoms to prevent a return to work. Lynch (1979) notes that disablement can become psychologically positive, extinguishing the reinforcement value of returning to work. Obviously, it is a complicated phenomenon in which numerous factors come into play. Schechter's (1981) review of data on severely disabled individuals indicates that individuals who had relatives financially dependent upon them and those with higher educational levels were more likely to work. Safilios-Rothschild (1970) also found that educational and income level are significant factors. Those with white-collar jobs and higher income levels are more likely to return to work than the poorly educated, unskilled, and low-paid.

Reactions to Career Changes

Workers who fall victim to secondary gain can be more easily understood when viewed in terms of the career changes they face and the impact of those changes on the workers. Involuntary career loss is a traumatic and devastating experience. "The necessity of identifying and beginning a new career, when the needs for security, self-direction, purpose, and future were being fulfilled in the former, may result in considerable turmoil. It is often accentuated by a grief reaction not easily understood by the individual involved" (Jones, 1979). While some workers may welcome a career change and even view the disability as a way out of manual labor, and thus look forward to rehabilitation, especially retraining, the majority of injured workers referred to and described by private rehabilitation specialists appear to fall into the former category.

Asher and Asher (1976) interviewed Dr. Lester Kesiser, a psychiatrist who has studied and written about compensable accidents. He implies that following the trauma of an injury that threatens paycheck, ego, and sense of worth and power, the person's and the family's expectations may shatter because of the loss of the job. The workers who are most affected by a work-related accident are those in the vulnerable trades, such as manufacturing, construction, and mining. Not only are accidents more common in these fields, but they also usually preclude a return to the job because of the physical nature of the work.

Workers who have received a substantial salary in return for their physical labor often become immobilized in planning to return to a labor market without their most valuable asset—physical ability. This may be especially likely in the case of an injured male head-of-the-household. Considering his age (usually mid-forties), his education (about ninth grade), and his previous work history (heavy labor usually performed outside), he is likely to be reluctant to consider starting over in a sedentary occupation that offers a substantially lower income. The anxiety initiated at the thought of giving up the comfortable lifestyle afforded by the high wages of physical labor occupations is often interpreted as the individual's malingering, but according to a rehabilitation specialist interviewed by Asher and Asher (1976), this is not usually true. The individual is simply grieving for his loss of livelihood and lifestyle. Lacking an education and faced with high mortgage payments, car payments, and school obligations for his children, the worker cannot make ends meet competing with younger entry-level employees in the less physically demanding fields. He may cling to the hope for a full recovery. Conflicting medical reports often encourage this behavior. Some try to go back to their old jobs, despite pain and risk of worsening the condition, because they see no alternatives to support their families in the style to which they have become accustomed. Lynch (1979) reports on a study of back-injured workers where 90% of a group of injured workers tried to return to work with 70% returning to the preinjury employer. Fifty-four percent of those people had to leave work, sometimes five or more times, due to aggravation of the injury. Of those returning to the preinjury employer, over 33% quit or were terminated within a year.

A study conducted by the West Virginia Division of Vocational Rehabilitation (1978) might help explain why injured workers in that state tried to return to their former jobs. While forty-six percent of the study's participants were coal miners, some of the results can be generalized to other populations of laborers. The study's findings were as follows:

- Clients prefer to remain in the industry where the pay is high and many benefits are available, even when told by doctors to seek other employment in a lighter work capacity.
- The client may be required to bid on lighter duty jobs as required by the union contract. Older workers with seniority may also bid for, and usually receive, the lighter jobs.
- Clients are reluctant to undertake training for new employment in jobs that do not match the wage scale of the industry in which they worked.
- Some clients distrust their employers and are confused by the conflicting information they receive.
- Educational background and former work history limit the opportunity for employment in other fields.
- Clients are reluctant to relocate. Many workers have lived in the area of employment all their lives. The industry is often the primary employer, and the area offers few other comparable alternatives of a light nature.
- Financial disincentives also include benefits from unions, such as pension plans and health benefits that have accumulated and will be lost if the worker leaves the union.

In cases similar to those described above, the workers feel it more productive to try to return to the former employer at all costs. When this doesn't work, they are then referred to rehabilitation, sometimes four or more years after the injury date.

In these cases, the injured worker often has little knowledge of the world of work. Eaton (1979) reports that the lack of occupational awareness alone is a barrier to rehabilitation. Fredrickson et al. (1978) reported that any adult facing these changes is apt to experience a lack of self-confidence, a reluctance to take risks, and an inability to make decisions, based on their limited awareness of occupational information. The clients described in this article seem to have limited flexibility, want instant success and prestige, and have difficulty in setting short-range goals. When a disability that precludes working in the former occupation, a limited work history, low education level, and limited transferable skills are added to this picture, it is easy to see how the injured worker's fear of career change far exceeds the "average" adult facing significant life change.

In addition, salary expectations are often unreasonable because of the lack of knowledge about other occupations. The sedentary, entry-level work that may be available often is initially rejected because of the high salaries manufacturing, construction, and mining occupations provide.

While facing these barriers, the client must deal with an insurance carrier who appears to be insensitive to the loss of high salary. Even though the carrier may have to make up part of the lost salary, thus adjusting total income, the worker may still look at the reduction in salary and feel a correlative reduction in self-esteem.

While experiencing fear, loss of self-esteem, pain, confusion, depression, and a host of other related feelings, the worker must consider rehabilitation. When the specialist is paid by the insurance carrier, it is easy for the worker to transfer feelings of distrust to the specialist, thus adding yet another barrier to a successful return to work.

Summary and Conclusion

Providing professional rehabilitation services to the injured worker is not a simple matter of providing job placement. Although a return to work is the desired outcome, the process of rehabilitating the injured worker is complicated by many issues and circumstances that must be considered if the practitioner hopes to provide high-quality, effective service. The rehabilitation specialist who attempts placement without being aware of the complexities that exist is likely to experience failure.

In reviewing the literature, the authors selected topics and issues that related specifically to the injured worker and also applied relevant concepts from the broader base of psychological and disability frameworks. Unfortunately, the rehabilitation aspects of providing service to injured workers is a neglected aspect of the rehabilitation field. Hopefully, the new emphasis on workers' compensation programs will alleviate the lack of data, research, and technical information on providing service to this population. It also seems evident that knowledge from other populations and related fields that may have direct relevance to the situation of the injured worker has not been adequately explored and applied. Issues of loss, lifestyle change, and counseling male clients are examples. It has been the purpose of this chapter to identify these issues for the consideration of the practitioner.

In the counseling of any individual, however, his or her unique circumstances and frame of reference must be carefully evaluated. Theories and research are only of value if they provide a greater understanding of the individual client and if they increase the possibility of successful rehabilitation. The reader is cautioned against rigidly applying theories to an individual case. Instead, the practitioner should use his or her evaluative skills and professional judgement to focus on those issues that have relevance to an individual case.

In examining complex issues, it is evident that the private sector rehabilitation specialist can and needs to assume a key role in the rehabilitation process. The specialist's role can be described as that of a synthesizer, coordinator, and catalyst. He or she must evaluate all aspects of the injured worker's situation (psychological, medical, financial, social, and vocational) as well as those factors which relate to workers' compensation law and litigation. He or she must coordinate the efforts of all parties and keep the client involved and informed at all stages of the rehabilitation process. The specialist must act as a catalyst by identifying the problems with the help of the client and other parties involved and facilitating the resolution of these problems through the creative application of services. To effectively carry out this role, the specialist must possess general rehabilitation skills, as well as having some specialized knowledge of medicine, law, insurance, and the needs of the injured worker.

The research indicates that simplistic labels of this population, like "cream of the crop" or as a group of "malingerers," only serves to discount the unique needs and dynamics of injured workers. Such careless appraisals fail to do justice to the complexity of the situation, overlook the challenges involved, and negate the need for skilled professional practitioners in the private sector. If private rehabilitation agencies are to continue to advance and prosper, they must be more than a placement service. They must provide the full range of rehabilitation services the client population they serve requires.

References

Asher, J., & Asher, J. Psychological consequences of on-the-job injury. *Job Safety and Health*, U.S. Department of Labor, 1976, *4*(3), 5–11.

Beals, R. K., & Hickman, N. W. Industrial injuries of the back and extremities. *The Journal of Bone and Joint Surgery*, 1972, *54*(8), 1593–1610.

Behan, R. C., & Hirschfield, A. H. The accident process II: Toward a more rational treatment of industrial injuries. *Journal of the American Medical Association*, 1963, *186*(4), 84–90.

Bond, M. B. Low back injury and industry. *Industrial Medicine*, 1970 *39*(5), 28–30.

Carlson, N. L. Male client – Female therapist. *The Personnel and Guidance Journal*, 1981, *60*(4), 228–231.

Chook, E. K. Criteria for return to work – Low back pain. *Industrial Medicine*, 1972, *41*(2), 32–34.

Conley, R. The vocational rehabilitation of workers' compensation cases: Facts and problems. Paper presented at the National Institute for the Industrially Injured, Rehabilitation Institute of Chicago, Chicago, Ill., October, 1976.

Conley, R., & Noble, J. Workers' compensation reform: Challenge for the 80's. *American Rehabilitation*, 1978, *3*(3), 19–26.

Eaton, M. W. Obstacles to the vocational rehabilitation of individuals receiving workers' compensation. *Journal of Rehabilitation*, 1979, *45*(2), 59–63.

Fey, S. G., & Fordyce, W. Behavioral rehabilitation of the chronic pain patient.

In E. L. Pan, T. E. Backer, & C. L. Vash (Eds.), *Annual Review of Rehabilitation*. New York: Springer Publishing Co., 1983.

Finley, M. H., & Lee, A. T. The terminated executive: It's like dying. *The Personnel and Guidance Journal*, 1981, *59*(6), 382–384.

Fredrickson, R. H., et al. Barriers to adult career change. *The Personnel and Guidance Journal*, 1978, *57*(3), 166–169.

Hirschfield, A. H., & Behan, R. C. The accident process I: Etiological considerations of industrial injuries. *Journal of the American Medical Association*, 1963, *186*(3), 193–199.

Hirschfield, A. H., & Behan, R. C. The accident process III: Disability: Acceptable and unacceptable. *Journal of the American Medical Association*, 1966, *197*(2), 125–129.

Hughes, F. Reaction to loss: Coping with disability and death. *Rehabilitation Counseling Bulletin*, 1980, *23*(4), 251–257.

International Rehabilitation Associates, Inc. Personal communication to the authors by Dan Davies, November, 1981.

Jones, W. H. Grief and involuntary career change: Its implications for counseling. *The Vocational Guidance Quarterly*, 1979, *27*(3), 196–201.

Keister, L. The traumatic neurosis. In J. J. Leedy (Ed.), *Compensation in psychiatric disability and rehabilitation*. Springfield, Mass.: C. C. Thomas, 1971.

Kowalsky, E. L. Grief: A lost lifestyle. *American Journal of Nursing*, 1978, *78*(3), 418–420.

Kübler-Ross, E. *On death and dying*. New York: Macmillan and Co., 1969.

Lynch, R. K. Vocational rehabilitation of workers' compensation clients. *Journal of Applied Rehabilitation Counseling*, 1979, *9*(4), 164–167.

Magora, A. Investigation of the relation between low back pain and occupation. *Industrial Medicine*, 1972, *41*(12), 5–8.

Parkes, C. M. Psycho-social transitions: Comparisons between the reactions to loss of a limb and loss of a spouse. *British Journal of Psychiatry*, 1975, *127*, 204–210.

Peterson, Y. The impact of physical disability on marital adjustment: A literature review. In P. W. Power & A. E. Dell Orto (Eds.), *Role of the family in the rehabilitation of the physically disabled*. Baltimore: University Park Press, 1980.

Ross, W. D. Differentiating compensation factors from traumatic factors. In J. J. Leedy (Ed.), *Compensation in psychiatric disability and rehabilitation*. Springfield, Mass.: C. C. Thomas, 1971.

Safilios-Rothschild, D. *The sociology and social psychology of disability and rehabilitation*. New York: Random House, 1970.

Sanchez, I., Workman, E., Morris, G., Miller, J., & Edelstein, M. *The California workers' compensation rehabilitation system*. New York: Macmillan, 1981.

Sawyer, G. The industrially injured: Proceedings of the National Training Institute. Chicago: Medical Rehabilitation Research and Training Center, *20*, 1976.

Schecter, E. S. Commitment to work and the self-perception of disability. *Social Security Bulletin*, 1981, *44*(6), 22–30, 37.

Scher, M. Men in hiding: A challenge for the counselor. *The Personnel and Guidance Journal*, 1981, *60*(4), 199–201.

Smedley, L. Workmen's compensation—A barrier to rehabilitation? In National Training Institute, *The industrially injured*. Rehabilitation Institute of Chicago, 1976.

Smoller, M., & Schulman, B. M. Chronic pain: Prevention through early intervention. *Occupational Health and Safety*, 1981, 50(3), *14*, 18–19, 21.

Treon, R. T. Private rehabilitation of injured persons: A plaintiff lawyer's perspective. *Journal of Rehabilitation*, 1979, *45*(3), 34–36.

U.S. Department of Education, Office of Special Education and Rehabilitative Services, Rehabilitation Services Administration. "Characteristics of persons rehabilitated in fiscal year 1979." Prepared by the Division of Program Data and Analysis, Office of Administrative Support.

Weinstein, M. R. The concept of the disability process. In P. W. Power & A. E. Dell Orto (Eds.), *Role of the family in the rehabilitation of the physically disabled*. Baltimore: University Park Press, 1980.

West Virginia Division of Vocational Rehabilitation. *Comprehensive vocational rehabilitation services for workmen's compensation fund claimant/referrals*. (RSA Grant No. 25–P–15508/3–03). Charleston, W.V.: September, 1978.

8 Use of Computer Systems in Private Sector Rehabilitation

Gary Golter

Introduction

Over the past 20 years, computer technology has responded to the economic, managerial, and technical needs of nearly every facet of our society. Its application to rehabilitation and other human services cannot remain far behind. The use of computers to assist private vocational rehabilitation practitioners on the administrative and counseling levels has tremendous potential.

In the business community it has been easy to visualize computers as money-saving aids to billing, payroll, and inventory control. It took many years of development for computers to move into assembly line operation and sophisticated decision making. Similarly, in rehabilitation and the related human services the full panoply of applications are just now emerging from the embryonic stage. It is most likely that in the next few years there will be giant strides in computer technology making its applications as indispensible to rehabilitation companies as it is now in industry.

Progress in this direction is already emerging in the public sector of rehabilitation counseling. During the past several years the demands to reduce the size of government and taxes at the federal, state, and local levels despite mounting demands for services have pressed government administrators to search for alternate and more cost-effective solutions. In this atmosphere computer technology is beginning to emerge as a means of agency survival. More and more state agencies are examining and testing its feasibility as a means of meeting the demands within the resources available.

This urgency is not yet evident in the private sector. As a result private rehabilitation firms are not moving into computer technology at the same pace. However, as the public sector begins to make some basic applications at first, and then moves into more involved and sophisticated applications, the private sector is bound to follow.

Both private and public sector organizations planning to use or presently utilizing computer technology are not taking full advantage of the available expertise that is in the field. The use of computer consultants is limited. In many instances, rehabilitation specialists without computer knowledge are making decisions concerning selection of software, hardware, and the application of computer technology. It is hoped that within the next several years rehabilitation practitioners will become more receptive and knowledgeable in this new technology, making greater use of available resources in the field and forging ahead with new and exciting computer systems for the vocational rehabilitation profession.

The History of Use of Computer Technology in the Human Service Industry

Until recently the use of computer systems in the human services has centered in five major application areas: management information systems, psychological test scoring, research information retrieval, client tracking or registration programs, and career information systems.

Management information systems have been in place in human services at state agencies throughout the country for many years. These systems use large scale computer hardware and process cost-accounting and client-tracking information. Informational resources for counselors expanded as federal, state, and county governments increased their efforts to develop coordinated, comprehensive, and up-to-date computer-based systems to provide information concerning new developments within the counseling field. However, recent cutbacks in federal funding have reversed this process, requiring the private sector to develop computer-based systems without the advantage of utilization experience in the public sector.

As early as 1968, publications by the American Psychological Association dealt with computer synthesis of psychometric data in vocational counseling. For a time, the federal government supported a Research Information System (RIS) in rehabilitation, which is described in a paper published by the Institute for the Crippled and Disabled in 1972. RIS had a central information base which evolved for the federally funded rehabilitation research and demonstration program. It was specifically designed to assess service alternatives and to be used by practitioners responsible for making decisions concerning service rather than formal research. Recent examples of computer-based research systems in the human services include the following:

- Accent on Information, a computerized retrieval system which provides disability information relevant to specific problems

- Adaptive Systems Corporation, a time-shared computer-based system which lists manufacturers of assistive devices
- Educational Resources Information Center (ERIC), a national information system designed to provide access to documents, books, manuscripts, journals, articles, and writings related to the human services and other areas.

In a collection of papers titled "Readings in Computer Based Guidance" (Oklahoma State University Research Foundation, 1970), the need for change in the area of career guidance and counseling was addressed, stressing the overwhelming amount of data which are insufficiently processed by traditional manual systems. Included in these papers were discussions of when these changes should occur and the alternatives for change. The report considered ways in which computers could be used successfully to support changes to manual career guidance procedures. Computer-based gaming is discussed as one computer technique that could assist vocational instruction and increase the vocational awareness of persons within the vocational exploration process.

Jim Norris (1976) stresses the benefits of utilizing computer technology in career planning at the community college level. He states that the computer should never replace the counselor; rather it should be used as an impartial tool to aid the counselor in the increasingly complex process of career counseling.

Reuven Kruger (1980), of the Research Utilization Laboratory located at the Woodrow Wilson Rehabilitation Center, discusses the use of information systems in vocational rehabilitation counseling. The following statement summarizes his position: "As our industrial based economy changes into an informational based economy, information activities will continue to permeate rehabilitation." The paper reviews the application of the new technologies, including computerized occupational information systems used to aid vocational planning. Systems reviewed include the federal government's Job Matching System (that system has now been phased out because of operational problems and lack of funding), the Michigan Occupational Information System (MOIS), and the federally mandated National Occupational Coordinating Committee organization (together with its state level committees). The degree of development and emphasis of public occupational information systems vary from state to state. For example, most public systems do not consider disability issues, thus permitting the selection of jobs with prohibitive physical demands for disabled users.

The Canadian Employment and Immigration Department has developed a comprehensive occupational information system (CHOICES). One privately developed career guidance system, the Guidance Information System (GIS), provides for the consideration of both aptitude and physical demand factors. Two systems have been developed specifically with rehabilitation in mind: The Ability Information Systems and VOCOMP (Computer Assist Job Matching Program), in which the counselor supplies data derived from carefully selected assessment techniques. (See the appendix to this chapter for where to write for more information on these programs and systems.)

The history of the use of computer-based information systems in private sector rehabilitation firms to date has been centered at a few large companies, such as International Rehabilitation Associates (IRA) and Comprehensive Rehabilitation Services (CRS). CRS uses computer technology effectively for case management, marketing analysis, billing, and a full range of financial applications. The CRS computer system can serve as a model in the industry for firms starting to plan for the use of computers to control expanding operations.

To review the history of the use of computer technology in the human service area, we see a great deal of research, a great deal of paper writing, a great deal of theorizing about the application of computers here and there, and very little actual implementation of operating systems. One of the problems is that the development of computer systems to support the public vocational rehabilitation effort has been centered at universities, colleges, and other nonprofit settings. The slow growth of computer technology in rehabilitation is associated with the traditional lack of experimentation by human service practitioners. However, since it is anticipated that new time-sharing services and microcomputer systems will be available for the rehabilitation industry over the next few years, the industry should experience dynamic growth in the use of computer technology in the years ahead.

Present Use of Computer Technology by Managers in Private Sector Rehabilitation

As with commercial corporations, the use of computer technology in private sector rehabilitation firms initially developed with accounting applications, especially to handle billing and accounts receivable. Computer technology was also applied to case registration systems developed to support marketing activities. The larger private firms were the first to develop case management and registration systems to provide a case catalog, current case status, and some rudimentary statistics to help the customer (the insurance company) understand the status of each case, why cases were not moving along, the costs to date, etc. The accumulation of the information by these case registration systems led to the availability of a great deal of case information for closed case statistical analysis.

Currently word processing is making its way into private sector rehabilitation firms as a way to assist in the preparation of the many reports that these firms send to insurance carriers and rehabilitation control agencies. Mailing lists are another early application because they can usually be processed on word processing equipment. We see in the use of computer technology by management in the private sector rehabilitation firms the same growth patterns, the same system priorities and use patterns that were identified for commercial corporations in the early 1960s. Private vocational rehabilitation management is sticking close to the standard accounting applications of billing, accounts receivable, payables, and general ledger, with some movement toward the management of case loads through the use of case management systems.

The recent availability of low cost microcomputers and time-sharing systems has opened the door for the use of computer technology even for the smallest firms. These firms can now take advantage of this new computer power for some standard accounting applications. A small business can now purchase a microcomputer system for about $4,000 to $5,000 or a computer terminal and printer for use with a time-sharing system for less than $3,000. Both are good capital investments. Computer hardware should be selected that will be expandable on a modular basis as processing needs change in the future. Initially a microcomputer can be purchased that will provide word processing, produce mailing lists for marketing, and allow a phased approach toward standard accounting applications available from computer manufacturers and software firms.

The microcomputer can also be used to be connected to a time-sharing service that offers a full range of specialized applications for vocational rehabilitation organizations and provides training and support services and the ability to expand into new services as needed. A company does not have to spend money developing specialized or custom software until experience is gained through the use of off-the-shelf software products or time-sharing services. Before any decision is made concerning the use of computer systems, it is recommended that the user's data processing needs be identified first and then a system implemented that fulfills those needs. As the user becomes more computer-sophisticated, the system can then be expanded to meet needs which were at first unforeseen.

Present Use of Computer Technology in the Counseling Process

Loughary and Tondow (1968) have conceptualized a three-level classification system for describing computer-assisted counseling systems. First level computer-assisted systems are information-processing tools. The second level goes beyond information processing and substitutes for counselors in performing certain tasks. These two levels are, however, totally controlled by the counselor. Computer systems in the third level are described as substitute counselors. Their significance is that their designer would attribute to them certain characteristics found in human counselors, such as privileged communication and privacy.

Examples of the first level of computer systems are the computerized test scoring, test result interpretation services, and research retrieval systems. The counselor administers one or several vocationally related tests to a client, sends a scoring sheet to a specialized company for computer scoring interpretation. Research retrieval services are usually large data bases of research information made available through computerized key word searches. Those applications expand the counselor's information handling capabilities and do not substitute for the counseling process. Level one systems illustrate the traditional use of computer technology by vocational rehabilitation counselors. Counselors typically do not hesitate to send tests to be scored by some remote computer nor do they usually have any resistance to using the computer as a research information retrieval tool if they are interested in obtaining research data for some purpose.

The use of computer systems at the second level, to substitute for certain counseling tasks, is exemplified by American Rehabilitation Management (ARM), a California-based private sector firm, which has used computers for this purpose for several years. Counselors at ARM use a computerized Job-Matching and Counselor Assistance System for occupational exploration and work history assessment. Level two computer systems have only surfaced within the last five years and usually address tasks associated with vocational planning. Examples of such systems developed specifically for the vocational rehabilitation industry are VOCOMP, and the Ability Information System.

Kruger (1980) describes systems that are rehabilitation-oriented and in which the rehabilitation counselor plays a critical role. VOCOMP, owned and distributed by Intracorp (the parent company of International Rehabilitation Associates), is a computerized job-matching system developed specifically for the vocational rehabilitation industry. It was developed and brought to the market by Innovative Software in 1977. Prior to that the only job-matching system that was operative in the vocational rehabilitation field was the HESTOR system, developed for the Goodwill Industries. The HESTOR system was tied directly to a work evaluation system and is based on the worker traits as defined on the U.S. Department of Labor's *Dictionary of Occupational Titles* (1977). VOCOMP brought the flexibility and the power of the computer directly into the hands of the vocational rehabilitation counselor. Unlike traditional career information systems that contained a great deal of information about careers but lacked the proper input definitions for disabled clients, VOCOMP is a system designed specifically to be used by counselors in dealing with disabled clients.

The selection of a career for a disabled individual is a complicated and time-consuming process which must involve both the client and the counselor. It demands a great deal of skill on the part of the counselor, who must demonstrate a knowledge of the physical and mental limitations imposed by a wide range of disabilities, as well as knowledge of the various jobs available in the local labor market and the physical and other requirements of those jobs. Under the traditional manual method, much time-consuming research is required in order to arrive at a vocational objective for a client. It is necessary to make sure that each client's special needs, abilities, and limitations imposed by the disability are considered in relationship to the demands of all jobs potentially available. All this must be done within the context of a fast-changing work world. Because of the complexity of these factors, it is extremely difficult to use traditional methods in vocational planning.

Thus, level two computer-based systems have been developed to assist the counselor in performing this task. Additional advantages of these level two systems are increased client motivation, simultaneous occupational prediction, and vocational reliability. Also, a greater amount of information is at the counselor's disposal.

However, level two systems have met with a great deal of resistance from counselors. Fear of loss of job and loss of interpersonal activity and unrealistic expectations appear to be the major contributors to this resistance. It is my conclusion after working with hundreds of counselors throughout the United States that a well-planned introduction of the technology coupled with workshop training, hands-on experience, and discretionary and voluntary use may eliminate much of the counselor resistance.

It has also been my experience that counselor resistance has lessened considerably in the last few years. With the increasing availability and general use of home and personal computers, computers are losing some of their mystique, and counselors are beginning to realize the advantages of using the technology. However, without full acceptance by counselors, computer systems cannot be improved to specifically meet counselors' needs. Counselors are needed as designers to help develop computer systems that will meet their exact requirements. This will open new career opportunity for practitioners who seek to improve procedures, methods, and the effectiveness of the rehabilitation profession.

Training appears to be the key to successful use of computers by counselors. Private rehabilitation companies installing computer systems for the counselor's use must treat training as a top priority in their planning. For example, when Innovative Software installed VOCOMP at the State of California Vocational Rehabilitation Department, training was initially planned for 50 to 100 counselors at one time to demonstrate the "wonders" of computer-assisted vocational exploration. That approach proved to be unsuccessful and actually increased counselor resistance. Not until counselor training occurred in a workshop setting with a small number of volunteer counselors did counselors start to use VOCOMP at any state rehabilitation office in California. In our work with other states, we have stressed the need for quality and individualized training coupled with available training support over the long term.

Realization of the third level, that of substitute counselor systems, appears to be many years in the future. However, some ground work has been done in computer-based interactive job skills training systems, such as Control Data Corporation's PLATO system. PLATO tutors students through a specific training program and provides some behavioral reinforcement and process monitoring. Many computer-based career guidance systems can be used by the client alone and do not require counselor intervention. We will deal more with level three systems as we look into the future later in this chapter.

Present Use of Computer Technology by Disabled Consumers

Use of computers by disabled consumers or clients has centered on computer-based training programs that teach computer programming. IBM's "Learning to be a Programmer" courseware and Control Data's HOMEWORK Program provide computer-assisted instruction that trains disabled people to program computers. Computer-based training techniques will be applied in the future to several other types of job training and counseling situations. Comprehensive Rehabilitation Services (CRS) has used the Eureka Career Information System to provide the client an opportunity to explore independently vocational alternatives. At the present time the use of computer technology to assist disabled clients has been very limited, but the potential is tremendous. The main barriers to increased use by consumers are the lack of available training programs and the need to adapt computer hardware for specific disabilities.

Future Uses of Computer Technology

This section deals with the future uses of computer technology in the private vocational rehabilitation sector. It will draw on examples of state-of-the-art technologies developed for the rehabilitation industry. This section will also describe some state-of-the-art computer programs being developed by other private sector firms and nonprofit organizations in the public sector.

Future Uses of Computer Technology by Managers in Private Sector Vocational Rehabilitation

Earlier, we discussed the use of client tracking or client registration computer systems by management. These systems are now evolving into full and flexible management information systems. An example is a management offered by Rehab Data, a company that provides rehabilitation cost control services to both insurance and private rehabilitation companies. This system works "by exception," that is, comparing active case status to predetermined time and cost standards for each type of service offered and identifying exceptions to those standards. As with a traditional case-tracking system, the user enters information about the case, but the Rehab Data system differs because it has built-in criteria for case service exception reporting. For example, if a job analysis is not completed by a certain date, the computer will list that fact as an exception.

This type of computer intelligence makes a tremendous difference between a static tracking system and a dynamic one. Once parameters have been established for the length of service time for each type of service, parameters can also be set for maximum billing to be allocated for each of those services. Exception criteria can also be developed from closed case experience by the computer itself, and therefore the computer can automatically update the exception criteria from time to time. This type of system can also help produce projections of cash flow by using the time and expense parameters to project when the billing for the service will occur. This is an example of the creative uses a computer system can be put to once intelligence is built into the system. As insurance carriers and other case referral sources become more sophisticated in the use of computer technology, more will include case cost management as part of their current claim management systems.

Of course, case management is just a part of what a private vocational rehabilitation firm needs to manage effectively the company's operation. Traditional accounting systems such as accounts payable, accounts receivable, payroll, and general ledger are critical ingredients to a full information system.

An example is a time-sharing system offered by Business Information Software, Inc., called the National Rehabilitation Time-Sharing Service (NRTS) (See the appendix for the address). NRTS offers a full range of services including billing/accounts receivable, accounts payable, general ledger/budgeting, case management, marketing analysis, mailing lists, counselor productivity analysis, and bonus calculation. Computer systems such as NRTS provide integrated management information systems which combine case management with the traditional accounting systems and also provide the user the capability to design their own report contents and formats. Therefore, when one wants to assess the level of business based on the line of business (e.g., workers' compensation versus long-term disability), a case management system should be able to provide that information immediately. An integrated information management system will provide feedback for decisions, including exception reporting and projections based on accumulated experience. It will be sensitive to changes taking place in the present business environment and will provide the capability for the user to design his or her own reports.

The service and cost benefits that result from information management systems are many. The reports generated can be very useful in marketing services by pointing out service results for each referral source. Since the system can be exception based, it can be very effective in managing the counselor case load. This will create a management atmosphere where the counselors are accountable for results because case information based on exception reporting is continually generated by the system. Cost benefits result from the most effective use of counselor and management time. In addition, case loads can be evenly distributed and cases can be assigned to those counselors who are most effective with certain types of clients.

Future Applications in Counselor's Use of Computer Technology

Decker and VanderWerf (1978) described the need for a computerized placement service. According to the authors, "A computerized system greatly reduces the time involved and can increase the number of job/client matches." Development of an employer job bank system was started at the Georgia Division of Vocational Rehabilitation, but unfortunately it was never completed. The concept of an employer job bank, containing open job requisitions, linked to computer files containing the qualifications of work-ready clients will be a major breakthrough for counselors placing disabled clients.

Some of the future developments in the area of computerized job-matching systems are illustrated by efforts underway to make job-matching systems even more effective for vocational rehabilitation counselors. They are (1) adding site modification and assistive device ideas to the data base and assuming the use of the device might compensate for a physical restriction in the job search, (2) providing automatic conversion of a variety of test scores as part of the client profile, (3) allowing the counselor to interact directly with the system through a computer terminal, (4) supplementing the *Dictionary of Occupational Titles* (D.O.T.) job description with more specific information from employers for both physical demands and other work measurements, and (5) integrating employer job banks with specific job openings.

Another new development in the use of computers in vocational rehabilitation is illustrated by two ergonomics projects conducted at the Fisher

Body Division of General Motors Corporation (Blache, 1981) and at the University of Michigan (Scott, 1981). Both projects used computers to determine the demands of a job as related to the physical capacity of a worker. Fisher Body uses a system called PLACE (Personnel Limitations Analyzed by Computerized Ergonomics) to place handicapped individuals and to evaluate the need for job modification.

Future Applications for Computer Technology by Disabled Consumers

Future potential uses of computers for disabled consumers are increasing dramatically. One potential consumer application is a computer-based communication network to be used by persons who are based at home by disability, allergies, phobias, or recuperation from an illness. This network will operate somewhat like a ham radio network, in which a confined person will use a microcomputer rather than a radio to communicate and interact with the community. A home-based person can be linked to an employer through the network and work at home as a computer programmer, key entry operator, editor, designer, and technical writer, and in many other vocations that can be accomplished remotely with the aid of a computer. The network will also enable home-based self-employment in the emerging professions of computer software development or as a data base designer designing special files useful to both disabled and nondisabled consumers. In addition, a disabled person will use the network to interface with service providers and support agencies. This network concept is an application of the present development of computer networks for home information retrieval and replacement of traditional printed materials.

Disabled consumers will also benefit from computer technology in the area of job training. An example of computer-based training is the Control Data Corporation's (CDC) PLATO System, which provides extensive training programs delivered through a computer terminal. Of course, the concept of job placement will change as home-based computers link disabled consumers to employers for several diverse occupations. Considering the ramifications of computer networking, a disabled client could receive services from a private sector rehabilitation firm at home through a computer network. For example, testing and vocational exploration can be accomplished with the client on one terminal and the counselor on another. Then once a vocation is selected, training can be provided through the computer terminal, including basic education skills, job-seeking skills, specific job training, independent living skills, and a variety of other training programs delivered via the computer terminal to the client at home. When training is completed, the client can then go to work using the computer terminal linked to an employer. Because the person is working at home, the overhead costs to the employer will be less.

Social programs can also be established through a computer network as the disabled consumers communicate with each other as advocates and relationships are formed. The service and cost-related benefits of the consumer-linked computer networks are many. The primary one is that a person doesn't have to be mobile for testing, training, or job placement. If local facilities don't exist for services, the services are delivered via the computer network. Another is that the computer-equipped home-bound worker enjoys low overhead expenses.

There are a few barriers to the future use of computer networks by disabled consumers. One is that the computer terminals may have to be specially designed to accommodate some disabilities. Another barrier is the possible elimination of the socialization process that occurs when people work side by side in an office. A third factor, the cost of computer hardware, is a barrier that is being broken by the availability of the low cost personal computers.

Guidelines for the Selection of Computer Technology Consultants, Services, and Products

The computer can be a powerful supportive tool for a private rehabilitation company. If improperly introduced, it can also be a source of disruption. As a company relies more and more on computer technology, management needs to understand how to purchase services and products that support the use of the computer system. There are many horror stories of companies being put out of business or placed in financial jeopardy because of poor planning and inadequate safeguards when installing new computer systems. So the selection of consultants, services, and products must be done with great care.

As a general rule, if one is considering an investment greater than $5,000 in computer technology, a consultant should be used to help make that decision. Computer consultants can be located through professional associates, personal referrals, the yellow pages, or colleges and universities. There are many computer professionals who understand the technology of computers, including computer languages, operating systems, systems analysis, and hardware and software applications. However, without some knowledge about the rehabilitation industry, these people don't do much good unless the company has the expertise to translate industry needs into computer terms that a technician can understand. One should try to find a consultant with several years of computer experience who knows the ins and outs of the rehabilitation business. Once the right person is located, references should be checked very carefully to make certain it is the right person. Whether the consultant knows the rehabilitation business can be determined, but others will have to be relied on to verify his/her technical knowledge. It can be helpful to visit a few clients of the consultant and have them demonstrate the computer system the consultant designed or the computer hardware the consultant helped them purchase. A telephone verification is too casual, and the contact will take the reference check more seriously in a personal visit.

Once a reliable computer consultant has been located, planning can start for computer hardware or software acquisition. The first assignment the computer consultant should be given is to review the company's need for a computer. This is called "needs assessment" and should include the following:

- A review of how the computer technology will be used to meet a specific need or goal of the company.
- An estimate of the cost to install a system.
- A brief cost benefit analysis.

Needs assessment would be equally applicable to the purchase of a word processor, microcomputer, the use of a computer time-sharing service, or development or purchase of a complete management information system.

If from the results of the needs assessment it has been concluded that the computer application is justified, it is time to do some comparative shopping. Remember computer technology is moving at lightning speed. What is not available today may be available next month, and what costs $10,000 this year may cost $2,000 next year. This means that when services and products are reviewed, it is critical that newly announced services and products also be explored. One should look past the sales representative into the research laboratory of computer manufacturers and software publishers to try to get a reading on what is going to be on the shelf within the next year.

Once new developments within the area of application have been determined, a comparison study of cost and performance (as reported by users), service reputation, service costs, and vendor experience should be conducted. A purchaser should be sure to contact and interview the references supplied by the computer vendor.

This is not a complete check list but an attempt to make a purchaser aware that a comparison study is an important step to take prior to the acquisition of computer hardware or software products. The proper consultant, system, hardware, and software are critical, and only careful step-by-step planning, study, advice, checking, and application will make it work. There are no short cuts.

Summary

Computer technology is advancing at a very rapid pace, but the application of this technology to the vocational rehabilitation process is moving very slowly. Factors that influence this discontinuity are the lack of proper computer training programs for rehabilitation practitioners and the absence of successfully demonstrated programs where computers have had a positive effect on the rehabilitation process and practitioners.

As we have seen, during the late 1960s and most of the 1970s, the application of computer technology to the human services centered mainly in research. The research cited in this chapter is mostly theoretical in approach; evidence of its transferability to practical applications is limited. In the rehabilitation field, the application of general computer technology theory to meet case management and counseling needs was almost nonexistent until the late 1970s.

In the second half of the 1970s, we began to see the emergence of the use of computers for the traditional financial applications, case registration, and tracking systems at state vocational rehabilitation agencies and eventually at large private sector firms. State agencies were able to move into computing before most of the private sector rehabilitation firms because of the volume of clients and the availability of central computers used by other state agencies. The application of computers in the service activities did not emerge until the late 1970s when career guidance, job matching, and employer job banks began to surface on an experimental basis.

The availability of small business computers brought computing power to the large multioffice vocational rehabilitation firms, but it was still mainly for financial applications. Billing, accounts receivable, and payroll were the applications first made by some private sector firms. Beginning with the 1980s, based on a growing interest in computer software products, it appears that the expansion of the use of computer technology into the service delivery functions has started. Case registration systems developed by a few larger firms to support sales programs are now being replaced by case management systems that deal with counselor accountability. Occupational information and job-matching systems are just beginning to receive attention as possible aids to counselors. Employer/client job banks to assist in the difficult task of job placement and the application of computer technology to job-site modification should also start to become realities.

The future promises many exciting uses of computers for managers and counselors of private sector rehabilitation firms, and their disabled clients. Integrated management information systems that combine financial and case management information with flexible reporting capabilities will enhance the control of service delivery by management.

Counselors will enjoy the ability to accomplish case-related research through computer terminals located on their desks. A full range of occupational information about job market trends, employer leads, training opportunities, local wage rates, assistive devices, and transportation accessability will be at a counselor's fingertips.

Disabled consumers will use computers to explore vocational alternatives, determine skills needed for a job, acquire training, and learn job-seeking skills; all of this can be done with the help of a computer terminal. Consumers will even use their computer terminals to work at home for a remote employer.

The rehabilitation profession will need to address the impact that this technology may have on the practitioner. The counselor's work will change dramatically as computer power brings the world to his or her desk. Counselors will spend most of their time counseling and supporting the disabled client through the difficult transition to a job rather than doing time-consuming research and report preparation. Accountability will begin to have more significance as computers help to control the many variables that now complicate the rehabilitation process.

Appendix: Computer Software

1. CHOICES, Advanced Development Division, Occupational and Career Analysis and Development Branch, Department of Manpower and Immigration, 400 Cumberland Street, Ottawa, Ontario, Canada KIA 059
2. GIS, Time Share Corporation, 2483 East Bayshore Blvd., Palo Alto, Calif. 94303
3. ESI-HESTER, Evaluation Systems Sales and Services, Inc., 809 West Madison, Chicago, Ill. 60607
4. VOCOMP, Intracorp, 985 Old Eagle School Rd., Wayne, Penn. 19087
5. Business Information Software, Inc., 19336 San Fernando Mission Blvd., Northridge, Calif. 91326
6. Ability Information Systems, E. 12411 Empire Way, Spokane, Wash. 99220
7. Rehab Data, Inc., 20121 Ventura Blvd., Woodland Hills, Calif. 91364

References

Blache, K. M. Applied ergonomics in manual materials handling at Fisher Body Division, General Motors Corporation. Paper presented at the Human Factors Association of Canada Conference, 1981.

Decker, R. S., & VanderWerf, S. Computerized placement service. *Journal of Applied Rehabilitation Counseling*, 1978, 9(2), 41–45.

Institute for the Crippled and Disabled. *A Guide to the use of the SRS Research Information System: Instruction manual.* Washington, D.C.: Superintendent of Documents, U.S. Government Printing Office, 1972.

Kruger, R. Occupational information systems and their use in rehabilitation. *Rehabilitation Literature.* Chicago, Ill.: National Easter Seal Society, 1980, Vol. 41, No. 9–10, 229–239.

Loughary, J. W., & Tondow, M. Computers as substitute counselors: Some possibilities. Washington, D.C.: American Psychological Association, 1968.

Norris, J. Community college career counseling and computer use, Sabbatical Report, 1976.

Oklahoma State University Research Foundation. Readings in computer based guidance. Washington, D.C.: Office of Education, 1970.

Scott, J. W. University of Michigan Ergonomics Project, Final report. Michigan Department of Education (Memorandum), 1981.

U.S. Department of Labor, *Dictionary of occupational titles*, Fourth Edition, 1977.

9 Getting Professional Training and Preparation

Carl E. Shawhan

Effective professional training is vital to quality service delivery. This includes preparatory training for individuals entering the rehabilitation profession in the private sector, as well as ongoing or continuing professional development. Training helps the professional to learn to do the job effectively, to maintain and improve performance in doing the job, and training helps solve performance problems that are identified. We must examine our individual and industry orientation. We must look to the history and development of rehabilitation in the private sector. We must identify who is served and in what setting. What are the services provided? And, what competencies are necessary to provide those services?

The Orientation

George T. Welch, founder of International Rehabilitation Associates (IRA), puts private sector rehabilitation in perspective when he says, "Insurance rehabilitation is a 'people business,' whose existence depends on how we service people's needs" (Welch, 1977). This means that we must care about the needs of each individual. We must ask, listen, and hear. We must design and provide products or services to meet the needs we identify.

Further, we must care *about* the individual, *not* for him or her. There must be respect for the person, for his/her interests and abilities. This is not rooted in charity or pity but in the value, dignity, and capacity we see in the individual.

Caring looks not only at needs but also at strengths and capabilities. Joe Batten (1981), a well-known management consultant, addresses this point when he describes the difference between judging and evaluating. Judging means to form an opinion and develop a mindset based on flaws, weaknesses, or faults of a person, circumstance, or event. Evaluating means to determine significance or worth by careful appraisal and study.

This approach to the individual, the organization, or event is a foundation of private rehabilitation. It is based upon identification and development of strengths and not upon a preoccupation with weaknesses and problems. What can the individual do? What are the transferable skills? What is the family support? What can the insurance carrier provide? How can the employer assist? What modifications can be made? What job openings exist? What products or services can I provide?

We expect positive answers to positive questions. We expect positives in ourselves. We look for and expect positives in the individual who is handicapped. This is what I call the "expective orientation" of rehabilitation in the private sector. It must be the orientation of the practitioner and the organization. It is the basis of our marketing and our strength. It is our integrity.

Professional training must be rooted in our expective rehabilitation orientation. If not, it lacks integrity and coherence. It is spotty and "techniquey" at best and at the worst is ineffective, wasteful, or detrimental. Our industry and its needed professional training are based on the worth and dignity of the individual, the value of meaningful work, and the capacity of our free enterprise system.

The Problem

The earliest efforts of rehabilitation in the United States were private efforts. The development and strength of the public vocational rehabilitation program have yielded significant benefits to handicapped citizens and have contributed to the development of rehabilitation in the private sector.

A brief review of the development of rehabilitation goals over the years reveals training needs for today. Early insurance industry involvement in rehabilitation in the 1940s was an attempt to achieve more effective medical management and cost control. This is still a key rehabilitation product or service today. Early practitioners and many rehabilitationists today come from the ranks of industrial nurses. They have training and experience in medical and psychological aspects of disability, in a team approach, and in communication with the disabled individual and with medical professionals. They bring a caring approach to the expective orientation of private sector rehabilitation.

As state workers' compensation laws developed the concept of returning injured workers to appropriate employment, rehabilitation services directed toward return to work (RTW) became another key product of private sector rehabilitation. Employer relations, job development, and job placement in the competitive labor market became critical job components for rehabilitationists in the private sector.

Rehabilitation counselors and evaluators from the public sector brought training and experience in coordination of medical services, vocational evaluation, counseling, and developing work-related skills. These people and other recruits from health care and human service fields brought a caring philosophy and value system which fit the expective rehabilitation orientation of private sector rehabilitation.

Rehabilitation managers began to look for specific characteristics of potential private sector rehabilitation professionals which seem to make them effective. A list of these characteristics might look like this:

- the necessary value orientation and concern about the individual
- enthusiasm
- creativity and imagination
- ability to sell oneself and inspire confidence
- ability to communicate verbally and in written form
- ability to market and sell rehabilitation services
- flexibility
- planning ability
- effective use of time
- ability to function independently
- ability to function as part of a team
- knowing one's limitations and working within them
- successful work experience (any area)
- commitment to one's own productive work and documentation of efforts and accomplishments.

Such a list has good face validity, yet much still needs to be done to look more critically at personal characteristics and training specific to particular work settings and products.

A majority of individuals enter private sector rehabilitation from health services, public rehabilitation, and allied social service backgrounds. The education and experience in the business community, in marketing, in insurance, and in job development/job placement with disabled individuals is usually very limited. William Emener and John Rasch express a strong need for greater emphasis upon the medical aspects of disability and upon job development and placement (Emener & Rasch, 1981).

Overview of Professional Training

The large private rehabilitation and insurance organizations are attending to the critical need for in-service training by developing in-house curricula, by working with academic institutions to develop and present tailored program offerings, and by providing paid professional internships. Some are expending 10% or more of their operational budgets to train new employees and to provide continuing professional development training.

Several master's degree rehabilitation training programs are responding to the need for more and better experimental training in the business arena. This is as important for public rehabilitation as it is for the private sector. Academic institutions such as Temple University, Pennsylvania State University, University of North Carolina, and Drake University have developed specific program offerings and have facilitated in-service training in the private sector.

Drake University, in response to the needs voiced by disabled individuals, business and industry, and the public and private rehabilitation sectors, has developed a master's degree program in rehabilitation job development/job placement. This is basically a marketing-oriented program with emphasis upon the needs of two kinds of consumers: disabled individuals and employers. It is experientially based with 17 of its 39 graduate hour credits based on work in the business/industry and rehabilitation communities.

The Drake University National Rehabilitation Job Development/Job Placement Program is a combined program with the College of Business and its Insurance Institute and the College of Education, which provides its curriculum development and rehabilitation expertise. The impact of this program is described by Gopal C. Pati in his management text, *Managing and Employing the Handicapped: The Untapped Potential*:

> Existing university curricula in the field of rehabilitation need to be reevaluated and revamped. Drake University, for example, has developed a master's degree in Rehabilitation/Job Development/Job Placement. The curriculum emphasizes (a) client development—"placeability and employability," (b) employer development—"attitudes, policies, practices, and accommodations," and (c) skills involved in job placement. The program heavily emphasizes labor economics and personnel management subjects. Such programs would take us a long way toward making the goal of independent living for disabled people a reality, not an illusion. It will also bring employers closer to the rehabilitation community, thereby resolving many perceived mysteries associated with the idea of rehabilitation. (Pati et al., 1981, p. 36)

Goals of Rehabilitation Curricula

It is important to articulate campus and field learning activities in the private sector. The learning in the classroom setting is applied in the field setting. It is tested and validated in the work environment. The total curriculum is, then, an articulated learning design of experience, evaluation, growth, and development. A key concern is development of individual values and "rehabilitation philosophy."

The next concern is with verbal and written communication. Verbal communication includes the ability of the rehabilitation professional to develop rapport with the disabled individual and his/her family. It means becoming an advocate to protect and to promote the welfare of the disabled individual and to facilitate the person's independence and return to meaningful work. Communication includes developing rapport with representatives of the carrier, with the physician and other medical professionals, with the attorney, with the employer, with the union, etc. Here, our integrity and our expective rehabilitation philosophy are critical. Verbal communication also includes our ability to market, our ability to be a consultation resource, and our ability to testify in court or before an administrative law judge. Communication means confidentiality and the necessity to safeguard information obtained in the course of practice.

Written communication requires technical writing skills. It involves understanding medical terminology and the ability to interpret evaluative information, particularly in the medical, psychological, and vocational areas. Private sector professionals must know the labor market, the jobs, and their demands. Report writing requires that the services proposed and/or provided be identified in terms of purpose and objectives. Professional rehabilitation activities must be fully documented and decisions and proposals assertively communicated. Proposals of services to be provided must be limited to those which the professional and the organization are qualified and competent to perform. The effectiveness of written communication by private sector rehabilitation depends upon clarity, brevity, and timeliness.

Many of the graduate rehabilitation training programs, including the program at Drake University, offer client-oriented training. These may include courses in orientation to rehabilitation, counseling, testing, occupational information, and medical and psychological aspects of disability.

It is important that rehabilitation courses or programs develop curricula directly related to rehabilitation in the private sector. Counseling courses must focus on utilization of vocational counseling and guidance and effective interview techniques. Testing courses must cover test selection and interpretation to include work sampling, situational work assessment, and vocational interest and achievement instruments. Occupational information courses should include theoretical concepts of vocational choice; trends, projections, and methodologies developed in job forecasting; conducting labor market surveys; and building a personal resource library and information retrieval system.

Medical and psychological aspects of disability should focus on the total individual and his/her environment with a vocational development model. What is happening with the individual at a particular time in life when disability is incurred? This question has significant implications for restoration of independence, rehabilitation goals and choice of rehabilitation services. Immediacy of rehabilitation referral and some particular areas such as cardiac, low-back, stress, and pain should be emphasized.

Knowledge of job development/job placement with the disabled individual is critical in returning the individual to work in the same job, a modified job, a different job in the same organization or to a job with a different employer. Knowledge of business/industry, employer needs, and specific job demands are crucial. The ability to relate with employers and to market what the individual with disability can do is a must. These are still very weak areas in the academic and experiential curricula in many graduate rehabilitation programs.

The National Rehabilitation Job Development/Job Placement Program

The Drake University National Rehabilitation Job Development/Job Placement Program stresses involvement in the business community. This means employer development, that is, establishing an employer relationship which is long-term and consultative in nature. It also means knowing employers, knowing employer needs, and knowing available jobs. Up to 85% of available jobs are in the "hidden labor market." These jobs become available as the private sector professional becomes an employer resource. Too often this necessary activity is limited in private sector rehabilitation because it may not be readily billed to the customer. Business training and preparation are vital to professional development and organizational development in the private sector. The Drake University curriculum stresses business coursework and actual experiential learning in the business/industry community. Highlights of the curricular offerings are described below.

Consumer Behavior. This course first surveys theoretical and empirical contributions to the knowledge of consumer behavior. The student is then prepared to investigate the consumer decision process from prepurchase to postpurchase activities. Emphasis is given to consumer behavior implications for marketing strategy.

Marketing Management. Administrative action is considered from the point of view of the interaction of the enterprise with its external environment, especially in the marketplace. Corporate objectives and policies are analyzed in terms of their impact on the adjustment of the business to competitive and regulatory pressures.

Human Behavior in Organizations. This course ties abstract theories of psychology and sociology to the actualities of the real world and the organizational structure. Person-to-person communication, fundamentals of organizational behavior, individual perception, organizational environment, and formation of attitudes and attitude change are stressed.

Personnel Management Techniques. This course acquaints the student with the tools, methods, and techniques useful in the staff function of human resource management. This includes development of practical skills in the recruiting process, the selection process, the placement (staffing) process, training and development, compensation, and equality of opportunity and affirmative action.

Wage and Salary Administration. This course covers federal and state laws affecting wage and salary administration, merit and performance rating, and budgeting with special emphasis on data processing relationships. It studies job analysis, job evaluation, rating and upgrading, and promotion and transfer.

Collective Bargaining. This course studies the relationship between management, unions, and workers at the level of the workplace. It studies the negotiation process and the law of contracts, grievance procedures, collective bargaining semantics, arbitration, conciliation, and mediation.

Applied Principles of Job Development and Placement. This course is the heart of the Drake University curriculum. The academic learning is articulated into field experience. It is designed to provide students with a basic understanding of the job development and job placement process with qualified handicapped individuals. Particular emphasis is placed upon a philosophy of placement; client evaluation, job readiness, and placeability; labor market and job analysis; job accommodation and modification; job development and placement; follow-up services and data utilization; resource services for the employer; and legislative and legal issues. The course reflects an underlying philosophy on placement:

> I submit that job placement is not salesmanship with emphasis upon the salesperson. Job placement is a marketing approach with emphasis upon employer needs and an intimate awareness of the capabilities, interests and limitations of the handicapped individual. It is the ability to meet employer needs with appropriate and qualified applicants. It is the ability to market and provide agency support services. It is becoming a vital employer resource. It is helping to meet client job needs. It is being a client advocate. (Shawhan, 1979, p. 73).

In the curriculum, marketing is defined as the disciplined task of creating and offering values to others for the purpose of achieving a desired response. It includes defining the market and defining our products and services. Job development/placement techniques are learned. They involve factors such as the types of contacts, the types and sizes of employers, determining who has authority to hire, and the steps of the contract process. Effective marketing means learning employer needs, concerns, and interests and learning to deal effectively with employer objections.

Placement is client centered and empowers the individual to manage his/her placement efforts. An effective philosophy of placement is to "do as little as possible, but every bit that is necessary."

The placement course develops human effectiveness skills and communication. This communication ability is critical in relating to client and family, employers, unions, service agencies, and insurers and with in-house agency relationships.

Vocational evaluation begins with determination of data needed, its collection and utilization. Individualizing evaluation is stressed. Study includes interviews, questionnaires, psychometric testing, situational assessment, and vocational evaluation systems (such as, Tower, HESTER, Singer, JEVS, VALPAR, McDonalds, MDWRS). Evaluation includes community, social and personal living needs, and competencies. Since past work history is the best predictor of future performance, the work history is studied beyond just looking for transferable skills.

Job readiness is an ill-defined term that has supposedly been a cornerstone of vocational rehabilitation over the years. Job readiness here is defined as the capacity to exhibit consistently performance patterns that will conform to those required by a specific job environment. The term may include not only employability, the ability to keep the job, but also placeability, the ability to get the job. Job readiness is job specific. Being ready for one job or even a similar cluster of jobs does not mean being ready for an infinite variety of jobs.

Client data, stressing functional skills and limitations, must be related to the previous job, the previous job with modifications, another job within the same firm, or a potential job with a different employer. This means effective job analysis and, where necessary, job modification or restructuring. It means being able to do labor market surveys and having an intimate involvement in the local labor market. The rehabilitation professional should belong to management, personnel, and civic organizations. It is through these relationships and the effective service we provide that the key to the hidden labor market is turned.

Other topics of the course are listed below:

- Development of self-placement behaviors, including client benefits, formal and informal information networks, job-finding client approach, job-seeking skills programs, client placement planning, applications and resumes, interviews and follow-up, job maintenance behaviors, and client rights
- Knowing the employer, including knowing the community, being

a part of the community, development of labor market data, utilization of labor market data, knowing the employer and employer needs, and job analysis
- Marketing techniques, including defining the market, defining our products/services, approaches to the market, meeting market needs and using placement services, and developing and using awareness programs for community, management, supervisor, and co-workers
- Job development/placement techniques, including types of contacts, types and sizes of employers, the gatekeepers, steps of the contact process, methods of contacts, employer needs, concerns, and interests, and employer objections
- Job accommodation, including modification and restructuring (human engineering and re-engineering of facilities, work stations, tools, and equipment)
- Job adjustment and follow-up services
- Alternatives to employment, including on-the-job training, projects with industry, rehabilitation facilities, and workshops, etc.
- Use of community resources
- Independent living
- Affirmative Action resource to employees and clients
- Wage and hour regulations
- Social and private insurance
- Union resources
- Rural versus urban placement services
- Placement systems and evaluation of placement process
- Time utilization
- Job development/job placement research
- Issues and trends.

Insurance and Insurance Rehabilitation. This course studies the development of private sector rehabilitation; the various settings, including hospital-based programs, insurance industry programs, private rehabilitation vendors, and employer-based programs; insurance and private rehabilitation; and the interviewing process.

Insurance is studied in terms of company organization, approach, and types of coverage. The roles of insurance company personnel are examined to determine where policy decisions are made about rehabilitation and where day-to-day rehabilitation case decisions occur. A comparison of some major insurance and reinsurance carriers is made. This approach is also used to investigate business/industry programs of self-insurance.

Study of the types of insurance coverage emphasizes workers' compensation and second injury funds, liability and casualty, long-term disability (LTD), and auto no-fault. The purpose of this study is to become a knowledgeable resource to carriers, claimants, attorneys, physicians, and others involved in the rehabilitation process.

Insurance rehabilitation is analyzed in terms of insurance companies, the self-insured, and the private rehabilitation companies and vendors. How an organization measures cost-effectiveness of rehabilitation is a critical issue. Types of rehabilitation services and benefits studied include medical management, financial and behavioral considerations, and vocational services with emphasis upon labor market survey, job development/placement, and follow-up. Testimony is a topic of study as are professional conduct and service delivery standards.

Again, the academic study can be articulated into practice through field experience and internships with business, carriers, and private rehabilitation companies. Examples include 3M and Kohler companies, Bankers Life, The Travelers Company, Crawford Rehabilitation, and International Rehabilitation Associates.

Future Implications

Professional training can be a key to getting the job done. It is critical in terms of quality of service delivery, credibility, and professional standards.

The private sector rehabilitation arena presently includes thousands of professionals providing various rehabilitation products and services to hundreds of thousands of disabled individuals each year. The private sector ranges from the one-person private-service provider to large regional, national, and international operations. It includes insurance rehabilitation programs, employer-based rehabilitation programs, organized labor programs, and hospital programs.

The private sector is beginning to develop into a unique profession. It is continuing to grow and develop, sometimes with limited direction and sometimes beyond the span of management control and quality assurance. The Insurance Rehabilitation Study Group and the National Association of Rehabilitation Professionals in the Private Sector (NARPPS) are taking leadership roles in addressing critical questions of professional conduct, service delivery standards, professional education training and experience, advocacy, testimony, confidentiality, business practices, and professional certification.

As we look at critical issues today, we often look to professional training as the cure-all or panacea. Robert Mager, the noted industrial trainer, has stated that about 80% to 90% of identified needs for training are, in fact, organization or management concerns. They do not directly relate to a need for training.

We must know what we want to achieve or where we want to be as a profession. We must be able to answer these same questions as an individual business organization and as a practitioner.

As we see and describe performance discrepancies, the first comment is often, "We need training." While training can be a solution to an identified performance problem, it may not be the problem. Mager and Pipe (1970) describe an effective way to analyze training needs. "Is the performance discrepancy really important?" If it is important, we must look to see if performance criteria are clear to the manager, supervisor, and practitioner. If so, is everyone aware it is important? Is it being measured? Is quality performance being reinforced, ignored, or even punished? Are there obstacles to performance that can be removed? Skill deficiencies in performing can be met through formal training before and during employment. We can arrange for on-job training, practice, and feedback. Training is vital, but it is not a panacea.

We are a maturing rehabilitation discipline. There is a need for formal academic preparation prior to practice and a need for continuing professional development. How can we best identify, facilitate, and support necessary training? The Insurance Rehabilitation Study Group, NARPPS, corporate organizations, educational institutions, and practitioners can provide leadership.

What is needed today is a national insurance rehabilitation institute. We need a focal point with industry-wide participation to address today's challenges and the opportunities and demands of tomorrow.

We need to better define our mission and to better identify and articulate our philosophy. We must look to even more efficient management of organizations and services.

What products/services are needed? Who are our consumers? What products do we wish to provide and what quality products can be provided? What professionals and professional training are needed? The present range of products runs from medical management to job development/job placement and return to work. They include industry/job related testimony and testimony in divorce courts. Products include employee assistance programs, wellness programs, alcohol rehabilitation programs, etc. We need an industry-wide market analysis or audit.

A national insurance rehabilitation institute can provide research and development to give us a better data base for program development and decision making. Such decision making includes a better understanding of who needs training and more specific data on what training is needed to ensure quality provision of identified products/services.

A national institute can help us effectively deal with questions of quality service delivery, certification, and standards. It can allow us to better meet needs of the disabled and potentially disabled workers. It can help us develop quality professional training.

We are a profession becoming. We have a positive, expective orientation. We reflect the value of the individual and the capacity of competition in our free enterprise system. Our success is based upon initiative, flexibility, and motivation. It is based upon early intervention, timely provision of appropriate services, and documented performance.

References

Batten, J. *Expectations and possibilities*. Reading, Mass.: Addison-Wesley Publishing Company, 1981.

Emener, W. G., & Rasch, J. D. *The 1981 Rehabilitation Education Survey*. Oklahoma State University, National Clearing House of Rehabilitation Materials, 1981.

Mager, R. F., & Pipe, P. *Analyzing performance problems or "you really oughta wanna."* Belmont, Calif.: Fearon Publishers, 1970.

Pati, G. C., Adkins, J. I., & Morrison, G. *Managing and employing the handicapped: The untapped potential*. Lake Forest, Ill.: Brace-Park: The Human Resources Press, 1981.

Shawhan, C. E. Counseling plus placement equals rehabilitation: Rehabilitation minus placement equals counseling. In *Job placement professional supplement*. Washington, D.C.: Job Placement Division, National Rehabilitation Association, 1979.

Welch, G. T. *International Rehabilitation Associates: Rehabilitation service manual*. Wayne, Penn.: International Rehabilitation Associates, Inc., 1977.

10 Getting Started

Marjorie Golter

So you want to start your own business! This chapter is intended to give some answers to the question, "If you knew now what you will know in five years, would you make the same decision?"

More specifically, the purpose of this chapter is to give some guidelines for getting started in a private sector rehabilitation business. It will begin with a discussion of the motivation for going out on your own as opposed to working for someone else. It will also discuss the importance of support systems (in terms of family, recreation, and advisors) and the structure your business might take. It will focus on what needs to be done and how to do it. The emphasis will be on the mechanics of starting a business and the problems involved.

To begin, there are usually certain necessities such as selecting an accountant and an attorney, setting up books, and writing a business plan. This chapter is designed to make you aware of the steps, not necessarily teach you how to do them. My aim is to share some of my experiences because I have gone through the transition from rehabilitation counselor to business person. The transition was difficult. It forced me to make many adjustments. Part of the process was the conflict between the rehabilitation counselor in me and the entrepreneur I needed to become. I have finally realized that by operating a business well, I have the time to creatively practice my profession. Running a business is like a game: there are rules to learn, and the quicker and better you learn them, the better the chance of success. Many of these rules I learned after the fact. It would have been easier if I had been able to anticipate events and base decisions accordingly. This luxury is not available to the beginner. Perhaps my start-up experiences will be helpful to others seeking to do it themselves.

Understand Your Motivation

There are many reasons why people go into business. One of them is simply boredom. "Many high level jobs in big business are crushingly dull" (Lowry, 1981). Owning your own business is a constant challenge, the antithesis of boredom. It is also an opportunity to test your ideas, to do things your own way, and to be your own boss.

The main reason my husband and I started Innovative Software was to make a new idea work (the appendix at the end of this chapter describes Innovative Software and its products in greater detail). We came from different professional experiences. By combining individual skills and training, we developed a new approach that we believed met a need that wasn't being met.

This brings me to risk taking. If you are not a risk taker, if you need security, forget the whole idea before you start. When we went to friends and individuals in related pursuits to test our ideas, we found very few willing to take risks, especially with someone else's product. But in business, the name of the game is risk taking. The risk isn't just one of "making it" or not, but rather making—or not making—each little step along the way. And there are literally thousands of these little steps; for example, meeting each day's expenses, being able to deliver next week what you said you could last week, and keeping your spirits up and thinking positively when you've just received "no's" from the ten individuals on the prospect list for the day. Remember, you must be able to sell more than your product to be successful in business. You must also sell yourself, your business, and your image of success. You are constantly selling, and the process of selling involves rejection. How well do you take rejection? Rejection will be 90% of your day—"No, you can't have that bank loan"; "Yes, I *love* your product, but my department manager is out of town, and when he gets back, I am going on vacation and then after that we are both going to the National Software Convention so. . . . " or "No, it is not okay to delay that bill for another ninety days. . . . " or "No, I can't type the proposal because I just broke a nail."

Of course, sometimes, someone is going to say yes, or you will have to close the doors, but most of your time will be devoted to working through rejections and turning them into opportunities. "OK, I can't have that bank loan, but can I have the loan if I put up collateral. . . . " or "The National Software Convention? Why, I am going to be there, and I can show our systems to both of you. . . . " or "How about ten days on that bill?" or "Here's some nail glue, and I expect the proposal to be finished in an hour!" This is an important concept to grasp. If you are a rehabilitation counselor and rehabilitation counseling really is all you want to do each day, do not open your own business because you will be doing less rehabilitation and more selling, negotiating, prodding, dealing with banks and administration.

The dream of financial gain is usually the motivation for going into business. Of course, the prospect of being independent and pursuing one's own goals and ideas can be important. The underlying drive must be to eventually turn a profit, to earn more than would be possible as a part of another's organization. The possibility of greater financial gain must be the enticement that leads one to take risks, to devote long hours, and suffer the challenges of administration, disappointment, and the chances of failure and defeat. Bedford of Bedford Partners, a firm with more than 30 million dollars of assets said, "The company's goal is to make money for the general and limited partners, not for some corporation" (Ferrell, 1981).

Many businesses fail. But, though there are failures, according to *Harvard Business Review* more than 85% of all small businesses show a profit (Lowry, 1981). When you hear of the increasing numbers of small business bankruptcies, it is important to remember that the total number of small businesses in the United States rose from fewer than two million in 1900 to 11 million today (Nickerson, 1981). The major reason most small businesses go bankrupt is undercapitalization. Contributing to the failures must be poor management and inadequate marketing and more often than not an inferior product not sufficiently tested before it is marketed.

When you start your business, you may need to take a substantial cut in salary, or "draw," but there is always the hope that as your company gets financially stronger, you will become financially stronger.

Vocational rehabilitation counselors going out on their own are motivated by the same factors as other entrepreneurs. They realize that by working for someone else, they are receiving a salary while their time is being billed out at a much higher rate. They want the prestige of doing their own work for their own firm. While working for another firm, they come to realize that they are doing their own marketing, thus building relationships that will carry them into a business of their own. Often what are not considered are the start-up costs and the delay between billing and collecting receivables. So what seems like a good idea can become a disaster if not carefully thought out.

Support Systems

The majority of rehabilitation firms in California in 1975 started as one-person operations and expanded as they became successful. The counselor then became a manager, marketing expert, and financial wizard, all in one.

Before making the decision to start your own business, you need to check out your support system. There will be many long hours, stressful days, and cash shortages, and unless your family is committed to you and your plans, you will not have the support you need. In addition, you will frequently experience tension at home.

Because my husband and I work together, we understand one another's tension, anger, and preoccupation. It is vital for your significant others to at least understand if not support you. We find it helpful to have a sense of humor and share it with our children. The issues and problems you are dealing with aren't funny; in fact, they are deadly serious, but incidents on a day to day basis are funny. For example, there was the time our bank account was overdrawn (because of the money we had poured into our business) and our house payment was due to hit the bank that day. My husband and I were ready to kill ourselves and anyone else who crossed our path. We called the bank to hear the bad news, and what we found out was that their computer broke down and their backup computer also broke down and thus the bank could handle no transactions that day. The next day the money to cover the account (money we had expected a week earlier) came in the mail. Well, you better believe we laughed! So make sure there is someone around who doesn't see things as half empty but rather as half full and on top of it all, funny! The president of *Ebony Magazine* has been quoted as saying, "If anyone talked about failing or not making it, I fired them" (television interview, August, 1980). You tend to fulfill your worst fears.

Of course, it always helps to have other sources of income, and you will need start-up funds or "seed money." A good formula to follow is to have enough funds to carry the business totally for six months and in part for an additional six months (Buge, 1979). If you are seeking investors, they would like to see you put your own money into the venture. It is better to use your passbooks or stocks as collateral for loans to the business and have the business pay off the loans. This sets up a good credit line for the business and leaves your personal funds free for future security and interest (Lowry, 1981). When you are figuring your start-up funds, double the amount of money you think you will need—and be sure to remember that if you think an invoice will be paid in 30 days, figure it for 60 or 90 days. The rehabilitation business involves collecting money from insurance companies and government agencies. Both are slow payers and, although you can feel confident that the money is always collectible, you can go out of business while waiting for the funds.

Another important aspect of starting your own business is setting up a rest and recreation program. You will be spending 24 hours a day, seven days a week, working and thinking about your business. It is crucial that there be some means for you to get away from it all. A good exercise program, a series of plays or concerts, etc., are good escapes. Since the job of running your business is so demanding, it is important to be in good health and to maintain that good health over the start-up years during which the emotional and physical demands are the greatest. If your rest and recreation includes your family, it serves a double purpose in including contact with your spouse and children during the start-up period. This is not the place to pinch pennies, as hospitalization and time off from work are far more expensive than getting some much-needed rest and recreation.

How about a Partner?

One of the early decisions you will be making is whether or not to have a partner. If you decide to have a partner, you might think about selecting someone from a different industry than rehabilitation. This is a process called "out-breaking" (Levine, 1981). Very often when all top management is from the same industry, such as rehabilitation, no new ideas are brought into the company. It may be that the financial or marketing techniques your partner brings from other industries can enhance the way your firm operates and give you an edge over other firms. Very often different temperaments facilitate good teamwork. One partner might be an outgoing person while the other partner is a stay-in-the-office personality. Both temperaments are needed. Partners can also offer one another moral support at different times. Of course partners need to complement one another. Remember, I said outbreaking mixes industries, not just areas of specialization. A marketing person in rehabilitation may not bring as much to a rehabilitation firm as a marketing person in toys. By crossing industries, knowledge is obtained from successful businesses which have been around for awhile, and you are adding a new dimension to your firm.

A partner can also supply what you lack in terms of money. Moreover, a partnership often has an easier time getting a bank loan than a sole owner. Investors also look favorably on a partnership. On the other hand, in a legal partnership, each partner is an agent of the other. This means that a check or contract signed by one binds the other. In addition, if one partner injures somebody while working for the business, all of the partners can be held responsible. A good rule of thumb to remember is that a partnership is only as strong as its weakest member (Lowry, 1981).

I think of a partnership as I do a marriage, and the relationship needs to have the same elements of trust, friendship, and working compatibility. If you can create that blend, there are many advantages to having a partner.

You Can Still Back Out

Before you make the final decision, keep in mind a few important realities. There will be no regular paychecks. Even when the business is doing well, the uncertainty of the future can necessitate leaving extra funds in the business so it can grow. Small mistakes can do you in. There is very little room for error in a small firm. Each mistake can be costly, and if it affects incoming revenue, it can cause your business to go under. Your mate and children won't see much of you. The days may be spent calling prospects, leaving the evenings as the only time for organizing the office and doing paper work. Finally, vacations and sick time often are very difficult to take. The expression "when the cat is away, the mice will play" is especially true in small businesses. If you are not there generating new business and overseeing details, the work will not get done as effectively. Of course, it goes without saying that a nine-to-five work day is a fantasy. Now, if you are still interested, read on.

Organization Structure

There are three ways to organize your business. You can form a partnership, with you as the general partner and your investors as limited partners. This is very attractive to investors, because their liability is limited to their investment, and the inevitable bank loans to the company can be a tax shelter for them. Limited partners have no decision-making power and assume no financial risk beyond their investment; they are only a source of funds. Depending on the partnership agreement, they can become or replace the general partners. The general partner or partners assume full control over the business and also assume full financial responsibility for its liabilities. If the business should fail, the general partner or partners are personally liable for all debts. Our firm is currently organized as a limited partnership. My husband and I are the general partners.

The second way to structure your business is to incorporate. A corporation eliminates most personal legal risk borne by general partners in a limited partnership and still allows for investors by selling a percentage of the business or shares of stock. A major potential disadvantage is the corporate tax structure. A corporation presently pays in federal taxes 17% of the first $25,000 of net income, 20% of the second $25,000, 30% of the next $25,000, 40% of the fourth $25,000, and 46% of the net income in excess of $100,000. Any income that goes to shareholders as dividends is also taxed. Finally, corporation losses are not tax deductible (though the sale of the investor's stock may generate a capital loss or a capital gain). However, most private sector rehabilitation firms currently are organized as corporations.[1]

Finally, a business can be structured as a sole proprietorship, which means you alone own your business. The rewards are all yours, and so are all the losses. Your home, your car, your bank account may all be at risk. A sole proprietorship is completely dependent on the owner's ability in every aspect of business (Kotter, 1979).

Board of Directors/Advisors

Depending on whether or not you are a partnership or corporation, you will need an advisory group or board of directors. As you gather your advisors, select experts in various areas and then really use them. You will be the one to assimilate the various pieces of information. Don't look for amateurs. Get information from people who have already demonstrated by their experience

[1]Tax laws permit exceptions to this tax structure (e.g., the "Sub-chapter S") under certain circumstances. You should consult an attorney or accountant about this before setting up.

and success that they know what they are talking about. Most rehabilitation firms are of the size in which seven board members are sufficient. In large companies, the board has more power and can hire and fire the company president. In small companies the president uses the board as an advisory group and consequently hires and fires the board. Obviously, the board must be so useful that the president doesn't want to lose them (Kotter, 1979). Typical board member backgrounds as reported by Hilley (1978) include manufacturing, law, investment, banking, and financing. Rehabilitation firms should also consider education and rehabilitation. Remember, you want people who have expertise in areas valuable to you and who complement your skills and experience.

Places to look for advisors or board members include the Small Business Administration (SBA), the local colleges, and consultants and executives of other firms. The SBA sponsors a group of retired business people (SCORE) who often act in an advisory capacity. There are many retired businessmen who, from their own experience, have a lot to teach to people starting new businesses.

Our firm's advisors come from the areas of law, economics, rehabilitation, gerontology, business consultation, telecommunication, and training. Each person offers fresh ideas and constantly helps us to expand our thinking. This process generates a business network of opportunities by exposing us to people outside our contacts as well as helping us develop an understanding of basic business principles. Our business is a computer software firm, which offers software products to firms involved in the rehabilitation industry. The two areas in which we do not have advisors are computer technology and counseling. We already have that expertise. Our advisors have been extremely helpful to us because they are not held back by the facts as we see them. We may be too much influenced by the issue most pressing at the moment, such as money, a specific contract, a personality problem, etc. An advisor can step back and advise us based on his or her expertise, without being biased by day-to-day operational issues. I believe a rehabilitation firm should have as board members an economist, a physician, an insurance company president, a financial expert, and a large manufacturing firm president. It has been my experience that rehabilitation firms are particularly guilty of inbreeding, and as with pedigree dogs, too much inbreeding reinforces weaknesses.

Your Attorney

Selecting your attorney is an important step. I recommend interviewing attorneys before selecting one. Find someone who has a background in business and who understands and appreciates your business. You will have to feel comfortable going to your attorney with questions. Attorneys are trained to represent and to protect you. On the one hand it is important to have that protection. On the other hand, freedom of action and the informality of a handshake can contribute to a business relationship. We had a large business deal sealed by a handshake, and our attorney desperately wanted to formalize it with a brief contract. We finally settled on a friendly letter that contained sufficient safeguards prescribed by our attorney. Our contract by handshake lasted 22 months and involved revenue of over $225,000. A formal contract would have offended the president of this company and probably ruined our deal.

You don't want an attorney with whom you can't get along or whose fees are beyond your reach. In such a case you won't consult when consultation and advice may be crucial. Find an attorney before you need one. Make sure that person is thoroughly familiar with your business plans, goals, and objectives. You may find that your needs are best served by a large, prestigious firm. However, your small, budding business may be assigned to a junior partner or associate. It may be that your interests can be better served by a smaller firm which can provide more personalized attention and the skills to meet your needs.

Before you start your business, design a few basic contracts that you think will meet the day-to-day needs of your business and that meet your attorney's approval. If you can afford it, have them printed using both sides of a heavy weighted paper. Leave spaces to fill in the specifics. Find out what the general rules are and follow your attorney's guidance and advice. In this way your attorney won't need to approve every contract, and you will save money.

Your Accountant

Your accountant will be as important to you as your attorney. Most rehabilitation firms don't have the volume for in-house accounting services or a financial officer, so you will want to locate a person who will serve as accountant, financial advisor and, depending on your size and expertise, bookkeeper, either full-time or part-time. If you are doing your own books, talk to your accountant before you proceed. He or she will instruct you on the most appropriate format and system. Your accountant can explain the basic accounting terms to you so you understand the general accounting principles for a small business. Also I recommend that you read a business accounting book. (Nickerson's 1981 *Accounting Handbook for Non-Accountants* is easy to understand.) Once you have a basic understanding of principles, you can then use your accountant for more than filling out tax returns and balancing your books. Your accountant can give you important financial advice.

You need to be able to ask questions regarding accounts receivable, accounts payable, the balance sheet, and other accounting matters. A good accountant can spot problems for you before they get out of hand.

When you are setting up your books, you must decide whether to report on a "cash" or "accrual" basis. When money is received, it is income, and when money is spent, it is expense. Accrual accounting reflects expenses as they are incurred whether or not a check is actually written. Similarly revenue is reported when it is earned whether or not payment is received (Nickerson, 1981). Accounting on a cash basis means revenues are reported when received and expenses when they are actually paid.

Accounting principles today usually call for accrual bookkeeping, and therefore, most businesses, whether service or sales oriented, report revenue when goods are delivered or services are performed. At the end of an accounting period, therefore, a substantial portion of the sales reported in income statements has not been realized in cash. In a small business this can lead a company to believe that expenses will be covered, when in fact, due to poor cash flow, the revenue may not be available when needed. You, therefore, need to know how much cash is coming in as well as what services have been billed which won't necessarily make cash available to meet incurred expenses. Thus it is imperative that accrual accounting be supplemented with a cash flow statement which estimates cash income and cash outflow at stated future intervals. In this way one can anticipate cash requirements and whether there will be funds available to meet expenses as they come due.

There are few companies today that account for expenses on a cash basis, as opposed to accrual basis. However, most firms want to know what expenses they have incurred in a specific month. A combination of accrual bookkeeping and cash flow reports will help a manager decide whether or not there are funds for expansion, new projects, or equipment. To get a clear picture of your business, both a cash flow statement of income and expense and an accrued statement of each are useful tools.

Locating a Bank

Once an internal operation is set up, you need to find a compatible bank. This is a crucial decision and often a very difficult one to make. Unfortunately, most banks will loan money only to a business with a proven success record. Moreover, they will not put a "value" on services you have performed until after they are billed. They also are put off by the fact that you are undercapitalized when capital is the thing you are there for. Before deciding upon a bank, talk to the loan officer with whom you will be dealing. Find someone who takes an interest in your business and sees the worth of your business as you do. Find out what the policy is regarding nonsufficient fund checks (will they call you before returning a check?). Will they give you a reserve line of credit? What are their requirements to quality for a loan?

One of the banking decisions you need to make is whether or not to keep your business and personal accounts at the same bank. On the positive side, your bank wants you to do this, and therefore, the placement of your personal account can help you earn "brownie points." On the other hand, you will have a better opportunity to manage your funds and more flexibility if your accounts are in separate banks.

The most important factor in finding a bank is getting a personal reference and introduction to the branch manager or to an important officer with whom you can establish a personal relationship. Then make that person your personal banker, if possible. A good reference and a good personal relationship are the most valuable assets you can establish with a bank, except a constant flow of large sums of money which tends to elude the small business person just starting out. Once you have the reference and have opened an account, try to maintain a modest daily balance and make all loan payments on time. If for some reason, a loan payment must be delayed, call the loan officer and inform that person of the reason for the delay and the date you will make the payment. This will assist in establishing credibility with the bank and enhance your standing.

If you take time to find the right bank and develop a good relationship with its officers, you will have a valuable ally. Financial planning, general accounting services, and answers to many business questions will be available to you. If you listen carefully, they will tell you what they want from you to establish a line of credit. A bank can also provide good financial advice and aid in establishing your image as a responsible, solid business executive.

Business Plan

Once you take care of these nuts and bolts of starting the business, you need to carefully write a business plan. This will serve to clarify in writing the objectives of the business, the financial projections, the market for your products or services, and the organization of your office and staff. It is my experience that the business plan should be completed before you start business. It will serve as a detailed overview of the nature of your business and keep you on track as you begin your marketing efforts. What often happens is that once you start working, the nature of your business shifts, and you must be aware that the shift is taking place. The business plan should be reviewed from time to time to permit an assessment of these shifts on a long-term basis.

The business plan, presented to your bank, or to marketing or public relations advisors, will give a clearer understanding of your business objectives. Many marketing firms will insist on a business plan before they will handle your account. The projections in the plan can serve as a guideline with which to evaluate projected revenue and expense. The sections of the plan describing your staff and their functions will clarify the responsibility of each person involved in your business and their position in the business's structure.

In your business plan you should address issues regarding the products or services you will offer. You should describe what you are going to do and how you are planning to do it. Be as specific as possible. "A rehabilitation firm counseling disabled clients" isn't enough! *How* are you going to do it? What are your *goals*? Are you trying to get people back to work or to close cases? Is your customer the insurance carrier or is it the disabled worker? What tools and methods are you going to use? These are issues to be addressed, and preparing a business plan forces you to consider them.

A Planning Technique

As part of the business plan I like to include critical path scheduling or PERT (Performance Evaluation and Review Technique) planning. In every new business there are major projects in which you will be involved, and PERT is an extremely effective technique to help accomplish this task.

PERT requires three elements, as described by Kroeber and LaForge (1980). First, the project must be broken down into separate components or activities. Each activity represents some part of the project that must be completed. Second, the order in which the activities can be performed must be determined. Some activities can be performed simultaneously while others can begin only when some preceding activity is finished. Finally, a time estimate for each activity must be given. Three estimates can be given—a likely estimate, a pessimistic estimate, and an optimistic estimate. The following terms are important in understanding PERT. They are

Activity: A subunit or component of the project.

Event: A milestone or checkpoint in the completion of the project.

Network: A schematic diagram that illustrates the activities in the project and the order in which they must be performed.

Path: A sequence of activities that is represented by connecting arrows through the entire network.

Critical Path: The path that requires the longest time to complete. Activities on the critical path are those with the potential to delay the entire project's completion.

Slack: The amount of delay that can be tolerated in reaching an event without delaying the whole project.[2]

I go into extra detail regarding PERT because I feel it is a very effective tool in planning and in managing various projects as they occur. My husband and I included it in our business plan in part to illustrate to our investors that we could manage the tasks required to get started and in part to plan to meet the financial requirements of the start-up.

One more comment about the PERT planning you will be doing: when you start adding costs to the individual projects, make a projection that you think is realistic. That projection should be labeled optimistic. Now make a pessimistic financial projection and assume that it is realistic. If your projections are correct, you will have money left over, but it is more likely that the pessimistic projection will be the realistic one.

Capitalization

"Every new idea in business has to bore through a stone wall of skepticism. The entrepreneurs who started Xerox, Polaroid, Readers Digest, and Ford Motor Company . . . were people with almost superhuman persistence" (Lowry, 1981). I inserted this quote more for my benefit than my readers', because I often need reassurance that those who "made it" faced the same frustrations that I am facing and that *there is hope*!

I have already discussed finding money from your partners and banks, but if you will be seeking investors or capitalization, here are a few pointers:

1. Don't use your own money. You will need any reserves you may have for personal resources. You would be paying extra taxes on your money, first on your income and second on the business's income if you loan your business money.
2. Plan ahead. Start preparing and planning for your need for investment money before you need it. If you are going to a bank, it is better to go when you don't need the money. This also applies to investors.
3. Line up 20 or more banks and talk to the presidents and loan officers. Banks like assets, not services, so you are going to have to take out loans for typewriters, computers, xerox machines, etc., rather than on invoices for services.

[2]This list is adapted from *The Manager's Guide to Statistics and Quantitative Methods*. For more information about PERT, see Kroeber & LaForge (1980).

4. Investors and lenders want to see a management team. Be sure you have one and make it part of your presentation.
5. Only approach a venture capital firm if you want a half-million dollars or more (Bibeault, 1982).
6. For small investments your friends, family, doctor, and lawyer are all people to approach, but you need to have a good business plan with reasonable projections, a good management team, and a product or service that has good prospects for making money.
7. Seek investors, be they bankers, friends, or acquaintances, who are interested in your business.

Market Research

Before you begin offering your services or selling your products, it is advisable to conduct some market research. Even if you are offering a standard service or product, market research can serve to expand or clarify your customer market. Whether you are selling auto parts or rehabilitation counseling, it is what makes you different from other companies that will make money. Marketing is the name of the game. You need to keep asking yourself, "What are we really selling?" "Who are our customers?" and "What do they want to buy?" (Lowry, 1981).

I think it is a good idea to involve your customers in the market research. Don't forget: you want to sell what they want to buy rather than what you want to sell. In 1975 when vocational rehabilitation for industrial injury cases became mandatory in California (where our firm is based), many firms were selling counseling while their customers wanted to buy job placement. Some of these firms were replaced by firms which sold job placement.

You also need to adjust to changes in the economy and in the attitudes of the population. For example, when we started our business, we said, "Hire the disabled, each person has the right to gainful employment." Now we say, "Hiring the disabled is cost-effective, and it lowers disability costs." To adjust to these changes, you need data. Initially the market research can be done by you, your customers, and your advisors. Your advisors and customers can give you a different perspective on your market and how to approach it. Later you may wish to hire outside resources to do the research.

Financial Requirements

It is a good idea to have a feeling for the time it takes your potential customers to pay. For example, most insurance companies pay on a 60 to 90 day schedule, and unless you are aware of this, you may get into serious trouble. Government agencies may delay even more. Often, if you offer government agencies a one-half of one percent discount, they pay within three weeks. This kind of information is important to have before you begin so you can plan discounts into your fee schedule. Most of your payables will be due in 30 days, and your payroll and taxes are due semimonthly. "When a company has an out of balance accounts receivable position with a big percentage of debts that have run 90 or 120 days, it has a serious financial management problem" (Nickerson, 1981). Before you have financial problems, it is good to know what your resources are. Your bank, of course, is one place to go for help. Sometimes it will lend on contracts but usually only after the services have been billed to the customer. Very often the bank will want to verify the invoices. The squeaky wheel gets greased! Call your customers and call your creditors. Try to bring in your receivables as early as possible, but be friendly and stretch out your payables as much as possible. This is no time for pride. Be honest, friendly, and push gently. Don't take no for an answer. Remember, "no" equals nothing, and anything is better than nothing.

Picture this situation, for example: A customer owes you $5,000. You call and ask for the whole amount explaining your poor cash position. They say "no," for whatever reason. Now you give them something. Be understanding and friendly and suggest a payment, let's say $1,000. They say $1,000 is too much right now, so you agree to $200 today and $500 by the end of the week and $500 next week. Ninety percent of the time you will at least get $200 which is more than nothing. If you do it a month before you need it, you will be ahead of the game.

Now for your creditors. If you are unable to pay promptly, call them before they call you. That is rule one. Some things like travel cards, gas cards, and bank cards are hard to manipulate. You lose something—a credit rating or the ability to charge. Other things such as the rent, your phone bill, and supplies can be stretched. You need to know how much and how to do it. Here is an example: The phone company sends a bill; if you don't pay it, the first month's bill will be added to the second month's bill, and both will be due in five days after you receive the second month's bill. At this point you can usually call the phone company and get a five-day extension on the first month's bill and a 12-day extension on the second month's bill. Sometimes it will require speaking to a supervisor. Now you are probably reading this and saying, "What does this have to do with rehabilitation?" and "My time is more valuable than that," and "How degrading," and "You have to pay it anyway." Well, it has to do with staying in business. We are talking about your financial resources, and occasionally the only resource you have is the time you can get by putting off paying your bills so you can collect your cash receivables. You may think you are trained for higher level things than this, but if you are not in business, you cannot be out there offering services.

Of course we would all love to be making so much money and managing finances so well that these things are not necessary. Be prepared! If the difference between success and failure is staying in business two more months, you had better be willing and able to make these calls and manage your funds! I am a rehabilitation counselor, and I know how to talk and listen to people, so I talk and listen to my creditors.

The other side of the coin is the management of a sudden windfall—instant success. That too needs to be analyzed and managed. In the rehabilitation business success carries with it the need for more staff and often more space. You need to be aware of the cost of hiring additional people and what your break even point is between the cost of delivering services and what you can bill. For example, how much can one counselor charge in billable work, and what are your direct costs from hiring that person? Maybe you will find that you make more profits by turning away some referrals. It takes careful planning and information to make those decisions.

One last word about money: the better you project your start-up costs, your cost of doing business, and your projections for work, the fewer problems you are likely to have. Whatever your initial projection for cash needs might be, double it. Whatever your initial projection for business might be, cut it in half.

Housekeeping

Finally you will have various housekeeping chores to take care of, such as establishing an office, getting phones installed, and making the forms required to do business. Make sure also that you have obtained all the necessary licenses and registered with the required government agencies. Before you order your forms, stationery, and cards, you will need an address. Therefore, you need to rent an office. You will want to shop around to find a reasonable rent, good parking facilities, and accessibility both in terms of highways, freeways, expressways, etc., and in terms of ramps for wheelchairs. If you are a service organization, it would be nice for you to find an office with ample free parking. Allow some room for growth, balancing the expense of moving versus the expense of unused space.

Compare the phone costs between private companies and the phone company. The private company phones cost more, but eventually you own the phone and pay only for the use of the lines.

You are ready to order your cards, stationery, and forms now that you have an address and phone number. It is worth the expense of hiring a graphic artist to create a logo for your firm. Your customers will begin to recognize your colors and logo, and it is a good marketing tool.

These tasks all sound so simple and mundane but can be expensive and time-consuming if improperly done. For example, installing a phone that doesn't rotate to another number can make it necessary to change your number six months down the road because you didn't get a rotary number. Plan ahead.

Summary

This chapter was designed for the rehabilitation counselor who wants to start a business. Throughout the chapter certain things, such as cash flow and planning, have been emphasized more than other points. That is because I have found that many counselors begin with the idea that starting out on your own means providing the service you always did, but now simply as your own boss. They fail to realize that they are doing a new job, which also requires certain new skills and knowledge. That new job is entrepreneurial. The better they do that new job, the more time they will have left to practice rehabilitation counseling.

As I mentioned before, most rehabilitation firms start as a one-person office and expand from there. The preliminary steps are all to be done before you start business, not as you expand; doing otherwise can be surmounted, but it is perilous.

The planning and thinking and decision making need to take place before you get started. Your advisors, bank, attorney, and accountant should be gathered before you start business. The questions of growth and procedures and forms and logo should all be addressed before you begin.

What often happens is that a counselor goes out on his or her own and, by the process of trial and error, finds out what steps should have been taken. How much grief and expense could have been saved with proper planning. In addition, the successful transition from a small (1 to 5 counselors) office to a large (20 or more counselors) office is often contingent upon the foundation that was built when the firm started. If you planned carefully, covered all the necessary steps, and allowed for growth in your financial planning, the firm can expand without major problems. The firms that began with the proper foundation are now profitable and growing.

Good luck.

Appendix: About Rehab Software

Rehab Software (formerly Innovative Software) started with financing from an investor group and is now a fast-growing company that provides computer-based products and services to commercial firms and public and private organizations that provide services to physically disabled persons. The company's clients include insurance firms, state departments of rehabilitation, rehabilitation hospitals, self-insured corporations, private rehabilitation firms, and a variety of educational agencies, among others. What Rehab Software offers is a unique blend of its founders' professional backgrounds and interests, fueled by a desire to give something of real value to the important field of vocational counseling for disabled people.

Not long after our marriage, my husband's background as a computer specialist and my training as a rehabilitation counselor resulted in a union of ideas that now is helping to put Rehab Software on the map, especially in California where workers' compensation legislation has opened wide many new opportunities in the field of services to the disabled—particularly workers injured on the job.

Our firm had start-up funds for the development of our product. We then had to rely on loans and revenue from sales to expand from California throughout the country.

One product, VOCOMP, utilizes computer technology and advanced data base techniques to provide an inexpensive and comprehensive job-matching and vocational-information system. Another product, RIMS, is a case management system similar to an automated diary system for rehabilitation services. It can be used for status retrieval and billing information. The customer can also design reports that would assist in their planning and marketing efforts.

Rehab Software is both a product development company and a service company. We do development and training, as well as provide services in many different settings dealing with professionals, clerks, and technologists.

Our company is located in Woodland Hills, California, with our central computer located in Encino, California. We have a small staff and utilize consultants on an as-needed basis. This way we are able to tap the expertise of leaders from various disciplines even though we are unable to afford these people on a permanent basis. In addition we have relationships with people in the field who market our products throughout the country. As we expand, we will be moving more and more toward a distributorship type of operation. We recently sold VOCOMP to Intracorp, an international rehab company, for use in their 110 offices.

Our future looks to the general employment market, to computer-based training packages, and to human resource systems designed for large companies, state agencies, and individuals concerned with employment. Employment issues will include outplacement, relocation of displaced workers, and career guidance for high-school students. The changing economy has been a challenge and an opportunity for Rehab Software. We see that as our constant task of the future—to keep up with these changes.

References

Bibeault, D. B. *Corporate turnaround—How managers turn losers into winners.* New York: McGraw-Hill, 1982.

Buge, E. W. *Administering the company financial function*. New York: Prentice-Hall, 1979.

Ferrell, K. 100 who made millions in 1981. *Venture, The Magazine for Entrepreneurs*, 1981, 47–51.

Filley, A. C. *The complete manager – What works when*. Champaign, Ill.: Research Press Company, 1978.

Kotter, J. P. *Power in management – How to understand, acquire and use it*. New York: AMACOM, 1979.

Kroeber, D. W., & LaForge, L. R. *The manager's guide to statistics and quantitative methods*: New York: McGraw-Hill, 1980.

Levine, J. Lessons learned when blue chips fail. *Venture*, 1981, 73–77.

Lowry, A. J. *How to become financially successful by owning your own business*. New York: Simon & Schuster, 1981.

Nickerson, C. B. *Accounting handbook for non-accountants*, (2nd ed.). Boston: CBI Publishing Company, Inc., 1981.

11 Marketing Rehabilitation Services

Kerry M. Boyle

Introduction

Private rehabilitation is a service (product) and as such must be purchased by a consumer. Our industry is somewhat unique, however, as the direct recipient of the service, that is, the client, is normally not the purchaser of the service. Rather, our customers (purchasers) usually are large insurance organizations having monetary interest in seeing that clients are effectively rehabilitated. The private rehabilitation professional, therefore, has a unique relationship involving both a client and a customer. This dual relationship poses some complex marketing challenges.

In discussing those challenges, let me begin by differentiating between the concept of marketing and the concept of sales:

Marketing. In order to effectively sell a product, an overall strategy or plan must be conceived so that the actual sales effort generates maximum return. Marketing activities involve identifying a group of potential customers, researching the actual needs of those customers, designing a product which will meet those needs, ranking the customers by their potential as referral sources, developing a plan for contacting potential customers, and installing an effective mechanism for measuring results. All of these activities take place prior to actually beginning to "sell" your product and provide the management framework which will hopefully produce maximum results.

Sales. Sales are the implementation phase of the marketing plan. Sales involve the actual contact with potential customers for the purpose of explaining the benefits of your service (as opposed to the many other services available) with the hopeful result being customer case referrals to your office. Sales is also the practice and development of the most effective technique for obtaining a positive response from your prospective customer.

Good marketing research and planning, without any kind of effective sales effort, will remain only good marketing and planning producing little business. Conversely, a strong sales effort with no overall marketing plan may result in some short-term gains but will eventually flounder as you begin selling the wrong products to the wrong people.

A combination of a sound and frequently updated marketing plan with an effective sales effort will allow you to develop a broad base of referrals, thus keeping your business viable and prosperous for many years. In the discussion that follows, the focus will be principally on the workers' compensation insurance marketplace, although techniques described would certainly apply equally to other forms of insurance-funded rehabilitation services.

The Marketing Concept

Preliminary Research

Your name is Terry Smith, you have a master's degree in vocational rehabilitation, and you have been working for a state agency for the last couple of years. You have heard that private rehabilitation is the field to get into but aren't quite sure how to go about it. One way would be to simply consult the yellow pages, call an insurance company, and say, "Hi, my name is Terry Smith. I do wonderful rehabilitation work and would like to have some business from your company." The response on the other end of the line might well be, "Well, we don't handle rehabilitation in this office, but would you like to buy a homeowners' policy?" If you have just quit your secure state job to go into private practice, a few phone conversations like this might cause you some mild concern. What is needed at this point is marketing research.

The first thing to determine is whether or not the state you reside in, or are planning to work in, has a workers' compensation law conducive to vocational rehabilitation. Workers' compensation benefits vary from state to state. While California has one of the most active private rehabilitation communities in the country, its neighboring state, Nevada, has very little private rehabilitation activity. Start your research by obtaining from the state workers' compensation administrative agency a copy of the current workers' compensation law—then read it. This is going to be a rather grueling task, but it is the important first step in getting a feel for your marketplace. Most of the law will make little sense; however, look for references to a "Vocational Rehabilitation Benefit" or "Earning Capacity" considerations as part of the overall workers' compensation benefit structure.

No matter how encouraging or discouraging the law seems to be on rehabilitation, keep in mind that what you are reading is only the broad framework of workers' compensation benefits as determined by the state legislature. The actual day-in day-out workings of the law are going to be further defined in "Administrative Rules and Regulations" or "Policies and Procedures." These procedures are written by the state workers' compensation agency in response to the legislative mandate. It is these inner workings of the system which will tell you whether or not there is really an active vocational rehabilitation market.

As an example, Comprehensive Rehabilitation Services, Inc. (CRS) was once considering entering a state which, after first reading of its law, appeared to have a very specific procedure for providing vocational rehabilitation services. After spending considerable time talking to those involved with workers' compensation in the state, I learned that there was no effective enforcement mechanism for seeing that the rehabilitation benefit was provided. Additionally, 70% of the workers' compensation business in the state was written by one insurance carrier, and that carrier had a very conservative attitude toward rehabilitation; that is, they didn't do it. In short, while the law looked good on paper, the market for workers' compensation rehabilitation really did not exist.

In order to avoid this kind of pitfall, your next step should be to go back to the state workers' compensation agency and obtain an appointment with one of the administrative law judges or other officials responsible for administering the law. Ask one of them to spend a few minutes with you explaining how the law actually works. Be persistent in seeking an appointment and don't be discouraged at all by the new concepts and buzz words which are going to be thrown at you. Remember, marketing research is learning about the market, and the more questions you ask, the more you are going to learn. Don't forget to obtain a copy of the agency's "Policies and Procedures" or "Rules and Regulations" governing the workers' compensation law.

Talking with the administrative agency's staff is an initial step in obtaining a picture of the role of vocational rehabilitation within the overall benefit delivery system. Assuming that the administrative agency personnel are somewhat encouraging, you must now talk to other parties to the system as different participants are going to have different points of view. Others you should consult include a minimum of two workers' compensation insurance companies, a defense attorney and a plaintiff attorney practicing workers' compensation laws, and a private rehabilitation professional practicing in the field.

A Minimum of Two Workers' Compensation Insurance Companies. Identify these through the yellow pages or ask your contact at the workers' compensation administrative agency which carriers they would recommend you talk to. When contacting the insurance company, ask the switchboard specifically for a workers' compensation claim supervisor or adjuster. Introduce yourself as someone new to the industry and be sure to indicate you are simply doing research. Most adjusters are willing to spend a couple of minutes giving you their thoughts on the frequency and viability of vocational rehabilitation within the state workers' compensation system. Be sure to ask the adjuster if there is a provision in the law for the settlement of the rehabilitation benefit. In many states, although there may be strong reference to vocational rehabilitation in the law and/or policy and procedures, the reality is that this benefit is often exchanged for a cash settlement with the injured worker. Adjusters are always interested in closing their claim files, so if a case can be settled with the approval of the administrative agency, they will often do so rather than going through the lengthy process of rehabilitating the injured worker. If case settlement appears to be the option most often taken when a person might otherwise qualify for rehabilitation, then your opportunity to provide services will be greatly limited. When talking with adjusters, remember that you are not selling anything yet but only gathering research data.

A Defense Attorney and a Plaintiff Attorney Practicing Workers' Compensation Law. Names of such attorneys can be obtained from the workers' compensation administrative agency or ask your insurance company contact. When talking with an attorney, simply state your intent of gathering data about how the system operates and indicate that you would appreciate his or her insights or suggestions. Most attorneys are willing to spend a few minutes with you on the telephone, although a face-to-face appointment is always preferable. Attorneys are an excellent source of information about how the law is really operating versus what may or may not be written in the statutes. States which have a high degree of litigation on their workers' compensation files, and where such litigation frequently includes rehabilitation, may be less attractive than states where the rehabilitation issues are not normally a part of the litigation process.

A Private Rehabilitation Professional Practicing in the Field. Through personal contacts or the yellow pages, locate a private rehabilitation practitioner currently operating in the field and ask if he or she will give you some advice as to the field's viability for you as a professional. Although you may encounter some initial resistance, I have found that most professionals are willing to share some of their experiences. A practitioner in the field can often give you valuable and accurate information as to the ease or difficulty of entering the business and the realities of practicing within the workers' compensation system. If you receive particularly discouraging feedback from your peer professional, remember that he/she may be trying to dissuade you from entering the field and thus becoming a competitor. Also keep in mind that a great number of private rehabilitation firms doing business in an area is a positive sign that there is an active market for this kind of service. Finally, never forget that someone currently practicing in the field may be your best source for entry-level employment in the area of private rehabilitation.

By now your picture of the workers' compensation insurance industry should be forming and the decision can be made as to whether or not it looks like a sound career opportunity. Additionally, and this is important, you should be getting a feel for the type of vocational rehabilitation product the marketplace is looking for and what they are willing to pay for that product.

Statistical Research

Having made the decision to begin working in private rehabilitation, the next task is to create a numerical picture of the marketplace. There may be hundreds of insurance company offices in your metropolitan area, and much valuable time can be expended attempting to make "sales calls" on companies that have little or no interest in purchasing rehabilitation services. Your time is your most valuable asset, and it must be used effectively.

Every state department of insurance publishes an annual report for the governor which lists all of the insurance companies doing business in that state and the premium volume they write. In many states, this document will also break the data down by type of insurance written, thus creating a ranking of insurance companies by volume of workers' compensation premiums they wrote in the previous calendar year.

In addition to the annually published commissioner's report, many state workers' compensation administrative agencies also publish annual studies on the number of injuries reported by various workers' compensation carriers. These publications are usually available to the general public at a nominal cost.

Statistical summaries like these are valuable marketing tools as they permit you not only to identify insurance companies that write workers' compensation insurance but also to group them into size rankings. The value of this analysis is that it allows you to spend your sales time with those carriers who write the highest volume of workers' compensation insurance and who thus are going to have the most potential for vocational rehabilitation referrals. If 20% of the insurance companies write 80% of the workers' compensation business (a not unusual ratio), you are going to want to spend the vast majority of your time with that 20%. Although you will certainly want to make some contacts with smaller carriers, it would be a mistake to spend most of your sales time visiting with companies who make very few rehabilitation referrals because of their low workers' compensation premium volume.

The list you develop should include each workers' compensation insurance company's name, address, and phone number. Next, organize them by groups—first into a group of the largest ten, then the second largest ten, the third ten, etc. This type of list will not only tell you where you should be spending most of your sales time but will also allow you to do some geographic planning so that running back and forth across town while making your calls is minimized.

The Marketing Plan

The marketing plan is the culmination of all the above research activities, and it is important that you commit to writing the steps to be taken in establishing yourself in the private rehabilitation sector. Your plan should include a statement of a goal or goals you would like to attain and the time frame within which to attain those goals. Although grandiose goals may be pleasing to the eye, try to limit yourself to practical accomplishments you would like to see your business attain over the upcoming twelve months. Once having decided upon three or four meaningful goals (too many goals will cause energies to be scattered), outline brief "action steps" which will allow you to attain each of the goals.

The action steps will identify specific daily activities necessary to meet your goals. As an example:

> Goal: Within twelve months, develop a referral base of at least three different insurance carriers each referring two cases per month.
>
> Action Steps
>
> 1. Create a list of the top 25 carriers, including names of claims personnel, in your geographic area.
> 2. Make a personal sales call on the workers' compensation claims supervisor at each of the above carriers.
> 3. Identify and begin attending meetings of the local claims associations.
> 4. Identify and begin attending meetings of the local insurance company rehabilitation nurses' association (if any).
> 5. Prepare a personal resume and a descriptive brochure outlining your services and fees.

Action steps listed in the marketing plan should have a completion date attached to them with a logical sequence to the completion of each activity. In the above example, step 5 should probably be changed to step 2 as you will not want to begin making sales calls until you have completed the design and printing of your sales brochure.

One goal which should be an integral part of all sales plans is the development of a broad base of referral sources in order to avoid becoming overly dependent on one or two insurance carriers for all of your business. One or two companies may be able to supply you with the cases needed to earn a comfortable living, but should you stop receiving referrals from one of these carriers, then you may theoretically lose half of your business. That 50% reduction may take a long time to replace, and you must ask yourself if you can afford to have a correspondingly drastic reduction in your income. The obviously preferable alternative is to work for a number of different insurance companies with no individual company representing more than 25% of your overall business.

At Comprehensive Rehabilitation Services, Inc., one of the marketing statistics I regularly monitor is our percentage distribution of cases from our various customers. If I see an overconcentration of referrals coming from two or three companies, e.g., 30% or 40%, then I know we must push for further development of smaller companies or acquisition of new customers in order to dilute that percentage. This is not to say that our positive relationship with those two or three accounts is not gratifying, only that good business sense dictates we not become overly dependent on them and thus risk serious financial strain should one or more of those key accounts decide to stop using our services.

Each goal you establish for yourself will have to have its own set of action steps, and you will find that some action steps may be appropriate to more than one goal. Development of the marketing plan will force you to clearly think through what it is you are trying to accomplish and apply discipline to your activities, thus giving you the highest probability of reaching defined goals.

The marketing environment is not a constant one; therefore, your plan should be reviewed at least monthly. Measure your progress against present time frames and, more importantly, evaluate the effectiveness of the steps taken to date. Although broad marketing goals should be adhered to in a twelve-month plan, individual action steps designed to reach those goals may be frequently altered as the needs of the customer or your success and/or failure dictate revised strategies.[1]

The most important thing to remember about a marketing plan is that its goals should allow you to reach a predetermined destination. The action steps or route you choose to approach that destination may change during transit, just as weather patterns might alter your route on a cross-country drive. The important thing is to reach the goal.

Selling Your Services

An old axiom in sales is that "nothing happens until someone sells something." As simplistic as this sounds, it is absolutely true. An insurance adjuster purchasing rehabilitation services will make a buying decision based on personal knowledge of the various rehabilitation service providers avail-

[1]A good plan development workbook is "The Short-Term Marketing Plan," published by The Conference Board, 845 Third Ave., New York, N.Y. 10022. Report #565, 1972.

able. The only way the adjuster can effectively learn of you and your service is by meeting you and that contact will rarely be initiated by the adjuster.

In making sales calls, the following steps need to be taken:

1. Have prepared, and professionally printed, a pamphlet or other handouts describing your services and your prices. Also be sure that you have a supply of business cards. (Around our company we have a standing joke that on any sales call we can always tell the marketing person from the counselor because the counselor is the one who forgot the business cards.)

2. Insurance personnel are busy people, so a preset appointment is preferable to "cold calls." Phone the adjuster you have identified through your statistical research described above, introduce yourself, and ask if you might have the opportunity to visit at a convenient time.

If you don't have the name of an appropriate adjuster, simply ask the insurance company's switchboard who is in charge of workers' compensation claims.

More often than not, your request for an appointment will be refused. Although initially discouraged, always ask if there is sometime in the future you can meet or if it would be all right for you to call back in two or three weeks so that an appointment can be arranged at that time. The adjuster will usually agree to a telephone recontact. Be sure to make a note to call that company back at the agreed upon time. In any sales activity, polite persistence will separate those who succeed from those who fall by the wayside.

3. When an appointment has been scheduled with the insurance company, arrive promptly at the designated time. Relax and open the discussion by asking a few simple questions about the company's operation, i.e., what territory do they cover, do they handle a large volume of workers' compensation claims, have they had a good deal of experience with private rehabilitation companies, etc. Although you don't want to play the role of an inquisitor, the more you can learn about their company, the referral procedure, and their attitudes about rehabilitation, the more effective you can be in describing your ability to meet those needs. Remember, your role as a sales person is not to simply tell them about all of the things you can do but rather to identify their rehabilitation needs and then explain how various aspects of your service can meet those needs.

4. After you have talked with the insurance carrier about their operation and needs in the rehabilitation area, tell them something about yourself and your services, keeping your comments succinct and to the point. Contrary to popular belief, effective sales presentations should involve no more than 40% of the dialogue coming from the presenter with the other 60% coming from the potential customer. The more the customer talks, the more you can learn about their needs, thus the more effective you can be in describing specific activities you as a professional can undertake to meet those needs.

5. At the conclusion of the sales call always ask your potential customer if they have any questions you might answer. Most importantly, ask if you might expect a referral from their office. Asking for the sale is probably the most important part of any individual sales call, and it is without doubt the most overlooked.

Several years ago, one of our counselors and I were visiting an insurance carrier, and an adjuster began talking about a most difficult case which would probably need rehabilitation assistance. My counselor politely answered all of the adjuster's questions about how the case might be handled and community resources which might assist the claimant. I stood there anxiously grinding my teeth waiting for the counselor to ask for the case as it was obvious to me that the adjuster was looking for professional assistance. Finally, I could stand it no longer and suggested that our counselor might be of direct assistance to the adjuster, and if they would let us review the file, we would take the information needed to begin a rehabilitation evaluation. The adjuster breathed a sigh of relief and gave us the case while the counselor looked at me rather sheepishly as she realized the adjuster had been hoping we would ask for the file. This is a rather obvious example of the need to ask for the business but underscores the importance of doing so.

6. A caveat: In addition to describing your services, it is most important that you present yourself as a professional. One of the most damaging things we can do in a customer's eyes is to engage in what I call negative marketing. Do not try to sell your product by downgrading or being critical of services or products of your competitors. Many insurance people have told me that they think little of a rehabilitation provider who uses this tactic as the competitor being criticized may be one they use and respect. Sell yourself based on the positive results you as a professional can obtain, not on the poor work your competitors may or may not be doing.

7. Finally, after the sales call is completed, it is a good idea to send the potential customer a brief note thanking them for their time and inviting them to feel free to give you a call should they have any questions or referrals.

Evaluating Your Sales Activity

After each sales call, you should reflect a few moments upon the kind of response received. Every call should be a learning experience. A sales call's success is not necessarily measured by picking up a referral as there is usually a one to four week delay between the call and the actual receipt of the referral. Although receiving the referral is the ultimate measure of your success as a sales person, there are other variables that measure the success of a call. Ask yourself these questions:

1. Do you know more about that potential customer and their needs after the call than you did before the call?
2. Does the potential customer now perceive you as a credible professional?
3. On your next call to that customer, will you have a better idea of the approach they might positively respond to?

If you can answer "yes" to all of these questions, then your call can be measured as a success, and over a period of time those successful calls will result in case referrals.

In addition to measuring the success of each call, you should also measure the frequency of calls being made. Depending on the goals you have outlined in your marketing plan, you should be making a minimum number of calls each day in order to get to all of the insurance companies you have identified as potential referral sources.

If your primary activity during the initial phase of your entry into this business is sales, then you should attempt to make at least four in-person sales calls each day. Although four calls a day does not sound like a lot, when you take into consideration all of the time spent on the telephone establishing appointments, you will see that it is a challenging, but not unattainable, goal.

Follow-Up Sales Calls

Once you have made a call on an insurance company, what do you do six weeks later when a referral has not been received? This will be the case more often than not, thus the follow-up sales call is very important.

After a period of several weeks with no referral being received, call the adjuster back and ask if you might see him or her again to discuss any files available for rehabilitation referral. The adjuster's response will probably be that they have not recently had any files to refer out but will keep you in mind. Reply that you appreciate the candor and that you will give them a call back in another three or four weeks. Most adjusters are agreeable to this type of follow-up. After several such follow-ups, either over the phone or in person, the adjuster may tell you that they really have no intention of using your service, in which case you reply that you will not bother them further and perhaps give them a call in six or eight months to see if the circumstances have changed. On the other hand, the adjuster may become weary of your follow-ups or admire your persistence and decide to give you a file and see what you can do with it.

One of CRS's customers today is a large insurance adjusting agency which refused to see us for almost two years. Every time we would call on this company, the claims manager told us that they were happy with the rehabilitation firms they were using and did not plan to use services from CRS. Undaunted, our marketing person continued to drop in on this claims manager every ninety days to see if they had changed their mind. After two years of persistent follow-up calls, the claims manager laughingly told us that he was now going to start using our company as we had been more persistent than any other rehabilitation company who had been calling on them. As mentioned before, this large adjusting agency is now one of our best customers.

Making follow-up sales calls is one of the more difficult challenges in sales as you often have little to say after having made the initial presentation. Follow-up sales calls require not only persistence but creativity. When you see the adjuster again, you want to provide him or her with additional or new information you might not have presented at the initial meeting. Sales literature indicates that the average sale is made on the fifth call on a customer, and I believe that this statistic holds true for our industry. If most of your peers make only one or two calls on a potential customer before becoming discouraged while you are willing to make four or five, then your probability of success with that customer rises greatly as you will be one of the few providers still calling on the customer.[2]

Service after the Sale

Receiving a case referral from an insurance carrier is not the last step in the ongoing marketing/sales process. The way the case is handled impacts on future referrals from that customer. In almost every situation where I have seen a deterioration of relationships between a counselor and an insurance carrier, it is because of a breakdown in communication. Insurance people are, generally speaking, not experts in the area of vocational rehabilitation, and you cannot assume that they understand why you are handling a case in a particular manner. It is important to the nurturing of an ongoing relationship that you maintain an open dialogue with your referral source, including written reports a minimum of every 30 days. Frequent telephone contacts, depending on the needs of the carrier, are also recommended. Insurance carriers will expect your activities to be well documented and presented to them in an intelligible and logical report giving specific recommendations for future activities.

When you see a need for a specific rehabilitation activity to take place, it is advisable to discuss the activity with the carrier prior to implementation. The carrier is both legally and financially responsible for rehabilitation, and nothing is more upsetting to the claims handling person than when

[2]Sample forms and formats for tracking sales activity and evaluating customers can be found in *Handbook of Sales and Marketing Forms and Formats*, R. Carlsen and J. McHugh, Prentice-Hall, Inc., Englewood Cliffs, N.J., 1978.

a rehabilitation professional discusses specific recommendations with a client prior to obtaining approval from the case handling adjuster. While your rehabilitation recommendations may make perfect sense, there may be legal or other considerations which the adjuster must consider. Thus, the adjuster must be continually consulted as the case progresses.

Since your referral source will be an insurance professional and not a rehabilitation professional, you cannot expect him or her to always recognize positive progress in your case. It is important that case success be "sold," so don't be afraid to tell your referral source about positive things that are happening in the case.

Additionally, you are not expected to be a miracle worker, and if you find that there are barriers to reaching realistic rehabilitation goals, discuss these barriers with the referral source and come to an agreement as to a mutually acceptable plan of action.

While your role as a professional is to help the disabled client, never forget that your funding source is the insurance carrier and the rehabilitation you are doing must conform to a well-defined legal-insurance environment. Always maintain an awareness of the boundaries of that environment.

Once a case has been resolved and, hopefully, closed, thank the referral source for allowing you to work with them on the file and ask for the opportunity to do so again. Keep in mind that the insurance professional is involved not only with rehabilitation providers but also attorneys, physicians, investigators, and various other outside professionals. Your work can be easily lost in the adjuster's busy world, not because of any lack of quality, but simply because of the number of people that adjuster must deal with on each file. Continually work to be visible to, and develop active working relationships with, adjusters so that they will keep you in the forefront of their thoughts when thinking about rehabilitation needs in their caseloads.

As you begin to work with more and more cases, it is a good idea to develop a closing summary sheet for each file. When work is completed on a case, jot down the pertinent information about the results, i.e., length of time the case was open, total billed, your impression of the adjuster's satisfaction with your work, the type of plan or other resolution which ultimately came out of the case, and any other details which you feel are important. The purpose of this exercise is to accumulate over a period of time a summary record of the average length of time you are keeping cases open, your average billing per case, and the type of results you are obtaining. A copy of a closing summary sheet should be maintained in each file and also kept in a separate file organized by insurance carrier. Such records will allow you to tell any individual carrier at any time what their average cost has been for your service and also the time frames and type of results you are obtaining.

Although we have previously discussed the importance of developing new customers in order to broaden your referral base, never forget that your largest source of new business is always going to be your current customers. Effective service after the sale and selling your successes will increase the probability of additional referrals from that customer and will strengthen your rapport with the adjuster.[3]

Unfortunately, I am aware of no publication which deals with the marketing of services in the area of rehabilitation. This is a new field and those operating in the field must study other bodies of marketing knowledge and adapt time-proven procedures to the peculiarities of our particular industry. For those interested in doing further research in this area, most business libraries carry numerous books and articles on the construction of a marketing plan, marketing theory and sales techniques and organizations.[4]

Summary and Conclusions

Effective sales of rehabilitation services are subject to all of the rules or principles which apply to the sales of any other product or service. The uniqueness of selling rehabilitation services is only that the "customer" we sell to will not be the direct recipient of the service.

As with any other sales activity, the process begins with sound market research to determine whether or not product demand exists and whether the service you intend to provide can meet that specific demand.

If the market research is positive, then a written marketing (sales) plan needs to be developed. This plan will outline the three or four major goals you would like to accomplish in the coming twelve months and enumerate specific strategies, including time frames, for reaching those goals. Only after doing your market research and developing a plan are you ready to "hit the streets" and sell your service.

Never assume that a potential customer knows what it is you do well and how your service might otherwise assist them. A critical part of the selling process is the use of questions in order to determine specifically what your customers' needs and prejudices are. A good salesperson should do more listening than talking because only through the use of questions and careful attention to your customers' answers can you determine what areas of your service should be highlighted for them. It is preferable to make sales calls by appointment and always to have an attractive piece of professionally prepared literature that can be used during the call and left with the customer. Finally, always ask for some business—"close the sale."

[3]For an interesting discussion of the pitfalls of a "high contact" service organization, see "Where Does the Customer Fit in a Service Operation?" Harvard Business Review, Nov.-Dec. 1978, 137.

[4]The American Management Association also sponsors numerous meetings and classes around the country, many dealing with marketing and sales. For a course catalogue write AMA, 135 W. 50th St., New York, N.Y. 10020.

Sales are not always made on the first call. In fact, general sales literature indicates that most customers do not give a company new business until the fourth or fifth sales call. Persistence in making follow-up calls to a potential customer is the one variable which ultimately separates the successful from the unsuccessful sales effort.

Once you have begun receiving business from a customer, it is a mistake to assume that they will continue referring cases indefinitely. Customers must be given ongoing attention to see that their rehabilitation needs are met and that they always understand the reasons for your success or failure on individual cases. Excellent casework will not always assure you of continued referrals. However, excellent casework in conjunction with positive personal rapport will create a high probability of a long-term professional relationship with that customer.

One of the persistent myths within our industry is that the nature of our professional services is so inherently good that they don't need to be "sold." This myth is based on the assumption (1) that you are the exclusive provider of this inherently good service and (2) that your customer recognizes the inherent good in this service. My fourteen years in sales, the last eight directly involved with rehabilitation services, have convinced me that both of these assumptions are false and that, although our product is most certainly humanitarian, it must still be sold to the potential customer. Sales efforts, in order to have long-term effectiveness, need to be well organized and specifically designed for the marketplace in which you are operating. Effective sales is a time- and energy-consuming activity but also a critical activity which can provide you with a great deal of professional gratification.

One last thought for those of you who may still not see sales as an integral part of your professional function. Once you have decided to go into business for yourself, mail out a brochure to as many people and companies as you can think of. Take out an ad in the yellow pages and be sure to tell all your friends and neighbors about this wonderful rehabilitation service you can provide. Now sit home and wait for the mailman to bring the cases and the phone to ring with inquiries. This will also be a good time to catch up on a lot of reading and sharpen up your resume because not much else is going to happen.

12 Planning Ahead

Jill K. Martin

In today's complex, rapidly changing and unpredictable economic environment, planning is one of the most vital parts of successful business management. Planning is, essentially, setting goals for your organization based on current and anticipated conditions and determining what courses of action will best help you attain them.

Developing a business plan, then, is problem solving. You must decide what you want your business to accomplish, evaluate the present situation, and outline steps you must take to get where you want to go. Good planning is also a continuing process. To obtain optimum results, the plan would provide for feedback from a variety of sources, periodic review to see how well it is working, and adjustments when necessary to reflect new developments within your company and the industry as a whole.

Business plans should also anticipate and prepare for as many potential problem areas as possible. In this way, the organization stands ready to act, rather than react, when crises occur.

A good analogy is the flight plan filed by a pilot prior to departure. The pilot must first know where he is, the condition and capacity of his aircraft, his desired destination, the topography of the land between his current location and the destination, and the weather conditions expected during the flight. Having determined these factors, he can calculate the best course for his flight and can estimate the amount of time and fuel needed for the trip. He then formulates a written plan which he files prior to takeoff based on the best information available at the time.

During the flight, a good pilot stays constantly alert to changing conditions as reported by his instruments, the weather service, other pilots, and his own perceptions and acts quickly to revise his operations and his plan as needed. For example, a strong wind may mean an adjustment in his heading to stay on course. A storm could mean taking more drastic action, such as stopping to refuel and delaying the flight until the weather clears. In spite of these minor or major adjustments, by referring to his basic flight plan, he knows where he is along the route at all times and can predict his safe arrival at the original destination with reasonable certainty.

The same is true with a good business plan. With it, the manager is able to predict and influence the future of the company, take early action to prevent problems, and efficiently handle unexpected developments while the company continues toward its established goals.

A simple example of good planning would be arranging for accounts receivable financing with your local bank.

> *Problem:* Let us say you are a manager of a firm which has seven employees. The company has grown from a single proprietor to this size over a two-year period. The company has one major customer who is a governmental agency and ten smaller customers who are insurance companies. The company is in a good financial position and has a large number of accounts receivable (that is, money billed to customers but not yet received). The major customer pays its bills regularly and usually within 30–60 days. The company has never had any problems paying bills or payroll. A budget has been prepared, and there does not appear to be any problem meeting the financial obligations in the coming year. You have some personal borrowing power but no actual financing arrangement with a bank. Unexpectedly, your major customer is changing to a computerized pay system which is causing major delays in the payment of your invoices. This is a temporary situation, but payments continue to be delayed even longer than the customer has informed you they would be. The day after tomorrow is payday, and you do not have sufficient funds to cover the checks. You do have sufficient borrowing power, and the bank is interested in making a business loan; however, the loan approval process will take several weeks.

This problem could have been prevented by good financial planning. Once a budget is developed and the financial projections developed, potential problems can be determined. Then, several banks can be approached for a financing package which may include a credit line based on the company's accounts receivable. Other types of financing might be arranged, such as credit cards, automobile financing, and/or term loans. During the course of the year, the company may not need to borrow money against its line of credit. But if it becomes necessary, the credit is available. Thus, by planning for the unexpected circumstances outlined above, a crisis is averted.

One of the largest problems facing most entrepreneurs is how to deal with growth. This problem is a common one in the rehabilitation industry, since the industry as a whole is young and growing rapidly. Many entrepreneurs do a good job of planning the start-up of their businesses but fail to anticipate the problems which come with growth, especially rapid growth. Therefore, it is essential to develop a plan which takes into account how quickly the organization should allow itself to grow and the problems that would develop with the growth.

An example of planning for growth-related problems would be developing an operational plan and schedule.

Problem: Suppose you went into business for yourself six months ago. You provided all the services yourself until three months ago when the referrals increased to a volume that required you to hire another counselor to work for you. You hired an individual with good credentials and provided some training. You have maintained your own caseload and marketing responsibilities. In addition, you now have increased billing, bookkeeping, and payroll responsibilities to meet, combined with training a new employee. You are working at least ten hours a day and frequently twelve hours. Today one of your best customers called with a serious complaint about the quality of services provided to two of his referrals, and he does not want to make any further referrals to your company at this time. Both of the cases are being handled by your new employee. Upon reviewing the files, you discover your employee lacks a clear understanding of the insurance system, has not defined case goals, and has not clearly documented his work.

An operational plan and time line would have prevented this problem. Such a plan would have identified in advance at what point you would need to hire additional help and how much of your time would be needed to adequately train and supervise the new counselor to maintain the provision of quality service.

Planning addresses a great variety of issues and factors affecting business. Because of the wide scope of planning, it is helpful to the beginning planner to break down the planning process.

The Planning Process

There are many factors to be considered in the planning process in order to obtain a clear, in-depth understanding of your business, your market, and your current and projected place in the market. This fact is particularly true in the rehabilitation industry because of the newness of the field, its current rapid growth, and the necessity of meeting state requirements which may change during the time period your plan covers.

If you are starting a new rehab business or are new to the field, you will find it helpful to review all current regulations and pending legislation prior to starting the actual planning process. You may also wish to talk with other professionals in your area to collect data on political activity in the state which may have a bearing on your operations. After you have done your homework on issues which affect the rehabilitation industry in particular, you'll be ready to review those areas which are inherent in planning for any profit-making small business.

Efficient planning should involve each and every part of your organization. Any area that is neglected can cause serious business problems, as we have seen in the two previous examples.

It is equally important that your managerial, professional, and support staff (if your company includes these positions) be involved in the planning process from the initial stages. Not only will their input provide information vital to the formulation of a realistic plan, but this team approach will also pay off by stimulating the interest and support of your staff in carrying out the formal plan when it is completed. You may also find it useful (especially if your company is a one-person practice) to request that a business associate, former colleague, or friend who operates a business review your draft plan to provide objective outside feedback on its clarity and feasibility.

Assistance in developing a business plan also can be obtained through publications offered by the Small Business Association and other government services as well as those privately published. (A list of recommended references follows this chapter.) Professional business and management associations in your locality may also offer written materials and workshops which you may find useful in the planning process.

The following are some of the specific areas which should be examined prior to formulating a formal plan. If you will take the time to write out concise answers to each of the questions—or at least carefully think each one through—you may make some interesting discoveries in areas you previously have taken for granted.

Market

In the rehabilitation industry, as in any other business, the more you know about your market and its needs, the better you can tailor your offered services to fit those needs and increase your share of available caseloads.

Before deciding whether to offer a full range of services or to specialize in a specific area or to determine why your business is not doing as well as you would like, take a long, hard look at the rehabilitation market in your area. What is the average annual expenditure for rehab-related services? What is the average number of potential clients per year? Is there a possibility of a large increase or decrease in the foreseeable future because of legislation? What is the state of the local economy? How will it affect the market? You also will want to identify your largest current and/or potential customers and decide whether you want to work for more than one type of customer (e.g., workers' compensation carriers, social security offices, attorneys, large employers).

Then get to know your competition. How many and who are they? Are they delivering the same services as you are now delivering or plan to deliver? Are your prices competitive? How does the quality of your services compare?

The final step is to make use of this data to determine what share of the market you currenty have, what share you can potentially hope to capture, and what steps you need to take to do so.

Product

Vocational rehabilitation is a broad-based industry. The scope of services you offer can be as specialized or as wide-ranging as you choose. However, to be successful, your choices should be realistic in terms of your market, available manpower, state requirements, and your finances.

After you have made the decision about which service(s) to offer, the next step is to decide exactly how you will deliver those services. A basic question to answer is whether you will offer individual services, group sessions, or both. Will your staff work with clients one-on-one throughout the case or as a team, handling different aspects of an individual case? Will vocational testing, as an example, be performed in-house or by a subcontractor? What method will be used—paper and pencil, work sample, or a combination?

You also will need to determine what resources and equipment you will need for product delivery. How will you establish contact and determine who the potential employers for your clients will be? Is a computer system more cost-effective than files for maintaining and updating current openings?

The questions and answers will vary depending on your size and your specific services, but think through all the phases involved and try to list all the areas about which you will need to make decisions. Now think of your current staff, their experience and expertise, and decide who will perform the duties defined in each category of service.

Manpower

The number of staff you employ and the skill levels required of each are dependent on a number of interrelated factors such as the kinds of services your company offers, state certification requirements, the volume of business you normally handle, and importantly, your financial resources.

As a start, when you are ready to hire staff or add to your current staff, the following rule of thumb can assist you in making those manpower decisions. To determine the number of clerical and professional staff your business requires, you first must determine the number and kinds of cases you have now and can reasonably expect to have in the near future. Next, based on your experience in the rehab field and on input from your staff, determine the average number of professional hours involved in processing each case. Multiply the number of cases by hours required then divide by 40 hours to determine man-weeks involved. This will give you a good estimate of the number of professionals you can expect to utilize full time at current and anticipated business levels. You can repeat this process to estimate the number of full-time clerical employees needed as well (hours per case × cases + 40 = 1 full-time position).

An alternative method for establishing the number of positions would be to determine the number of projected open files and apply your company's staffing ratios. This method is less precise and requires some experience and expertise to determine the ratios. An example of how this might work can be seen in Table 12–1. Obviously, no one works at full capacity every hour on the job, and allowances must also be made for sick leave, vacations, training, and other factors. So use these figures as a guide, not a hard and fast rule.

You may also want to consider part-time or temporary employees for certain types of work involved in your calculations (e.g., weekly workshops or clerical relief during holiday periods). If your figures indicate too many hours for three employees, but not enough for four, a part-time employee may be the solution.

You also will need to consider the number and kind of managerial and administrative support staff needed for your specific operations. Managerial staff, including yourself, will be involved in financial and operational planning as well as in overall supervision. Administrative support staff will include those who perform personnel functions, bookkeeping/accounting activities, and purchasing. Depending on your company size and your expertise,

Table 12–1. Estimating Professional and Clerical Staff Positions

	Nov.	*Dec.*
Active cases on first of month	180	185
Cases to be opened (add)	30	20
Cases to be closed (subtract)	25	25
Professional staff case loads (at 20 to 25 cases per staff)	9.25 high/ 7.4 low	9.0 high/ 7.2 low
Approximate average of professional case loads	8	8
Clerical staff case loads (at 100 to 125 cases per staff)	1.85 high/ 1.48 low	1.8 high/ 1.44 low
Approximate average of clerical case loads	1.5	1.5

Therefore, 8 professional staff and 1.5 clerical staff are needed.

you may choose to perform some or all of these activities yourself or hire full- or part-time staff for each or a combination of them. As an alternative, you might want to consider the use of subcontractors for some of the professional and support services, either individuals or companies. For example, if your operations do not require enough psychological and vocational testing to support a full- or part-time employee, you may wish to contract with a firm specializing in testing to perform these services.

For another example, you may find it more cost-effective to use a professional accountant paid on an hourly basis rather than hiring a full-time bookkeeper/accountant.

Another important manpower consideration is the skill levels you require in meeting company needs. As part of a regulated and specialized industry, your staff must have the education, experience, credentials, and other qualifications to maintain state certification in your location. Become familiar with those requirements and the certification process, and try to find out if legislation or other action is likely to change them in the foreseeable future.

You also will need to consider the particular skills required to deliver the services your company offers. Is there a sufficient pool of trained professionals in your community or will you need more broadly based recruiting? How much on-the-job training do you want to provide? Who will do the training? Do you need generalists or specialists such as work evaluators, job developers, or psychometrists? The answers to these questions depend on your specific company and the state or states in which you do business, so think it over carefully.

Last, but far from least, all these manpower decisions must be made based on the financial realities of your business. After you have done your homework to analyze the above factors and determined typical salaries in your area for the positions you want to fill, you may need to review your proposed staffing and make adjustments, if necessary, based on your financial resources.

Facilities

The size, type, and location of your facilities depend on a number of factors, for example, the territory you cover in your operations and the kind of services you offer. Do you have the proper facilities to support your goals? Here are some more questions you should ask yourself about your facilities:

- Are your offices centrally located in your service area? Are they easily accessible by public transportation? Is there adequate parking?
- Many of the clients you serve as a rehabilitation business may have minor or major disabilities which limit mobility. Is there wheelchair access? Elevator service?

- Are your offices properly laid out to provide adequate space for your staff and equipment? To provide privacy for client conferences?
- Do you have flexibility for expansion? To meet varying work loads?
- Based on your specific needs and financial operations, is it more advisable to rent, lease, or buy? Why?

Financial Operations

No plan can work without sufficient financial resources available at the right time to support planned activities necessary to accomplish your goals and objectives. That would be equivalent to taking off in the plane we have been discussing with no fuel in the tanks. A healthy business must have a healthy cash flow. This means that accounts receivable (income to you from all sources) must at least equal accounts payable (payments from you to all suppliers) plus operating expenses (salaries, taxes, social security, workers' compensation, equipment, rent/lease/purchase payments, etc.). This income must also produce sufficient cash reserves to meet periodic and/or long-term expenses. It is important that incoming cash not only be sufficient in overall amount, it must also be received in a timely fashion to ensure that you have money on hand when you need it to pay expenses in full and on time. Planning ways to maintain a healthy cash flow puts you in control of your financial stability and profitability. Ask yourself these questions:

- Do certain customers pay on different schedules than others, i.e., federal government versus private insurance carriers? When and why? Can these schedules be changed to better meet your cash flow needs? Would changing your billing schedule result in quicker payment?
- Is your monthly billing equal to monthly expenses? If not, how can you increase billings or decrease expenses? How will you make up the deficit until then?
- Are your invoices being paid within the time you allot for payment? If not, why not? Are you consistently following up on delinquent accounts? How? Is this method working? How can you improve your method?

Another important area of financial operations is your borrowing power. The appropriate time to determine your credit worthiness is before you need a loan to meet emergency expenses, to make major purchases, or to carry out expansion plans.

After you have selected a bank or other financial institution for your business account, get to know your financial officer. Ask about long- and short-term loan requirements and make sure your company qualifies. Is your credit rating acceptable? How can you improve it? Can your bookkeeping methods quickly and easily produce required information?

You may also want to arrange a line of credit with your banking institution based on your accounts receivable or overall profitability. This means, in effect, that you go through all the steps necessary to obtain a loan in an amount agreed upon, but you don't actually borrow funds until you need the money. If and when you do, receiving the funds usually requires only a phone call to the loan officer who will then place part or all of the agreed upon amount in your business account. No interest is charged until the money is received, and the percentage rate is usually determined by the rate in effect on that date. The term of the loan will be that worked out by you and the loan officer earlier.

Again, planning ahead can save you time and effort and in many cases can help you avoid a financial emergency that could adversely affect your credit rating or severely affect your daily operations.

Regulatory/Legislative

It is imperative to keep yourself well-informed on the operations of the state government in your location. After regulations adversely affecting your business are already in effect, it is very difficult to try to change them. Testifying at hearings concerning laws, rules, and regulations affecting your industry is important. Depending again on your specific location, you may want to work to change legislation or regulations either through your individual efforts or by joining other providers in lobbying efforts.

The Formal Plan

Now that you have reviewed all areas of operation, thought over the elements involved in formulating a plan, and made some preliminary notes, it is time to put the plan in writing. With a written plan, managerial, professional, and clerical staff have a clear and uniform understanding of the company and the course of action they will be expected to take to achieve the company's goals.

An effective business plan should include the following:

- Objectives: long-term and short-term;
- Strategies for achieving those objectives;
- Planned activities required by the strategies;
- Staff assignments for each activity;
- Timetables for completion of each task;
- A budget for each strategy;
- Target dates for review and updating of the plan to reflect changing conditions;

- And, perhaps the most important element, the cooperation and support of every individual in the company to achieve the stated objectives.

There may be separate plans for each objective or for each area of operation. Try to be as specific and realistic as possible in each area. The final step in the planning process is the integration of individual plans into a master plan for your organization.

Ready for takeoff?

Step 1. Define the overall purpose of your business. (What is the purpose of this flight?) What is your philosophy and how does it fit with the industry? Are you generalists or specialists?

Step 2. Assess the current problems and opportunities of your business. (Is your craft an airliner or a puddle jumper?) What are the capabilities of your staff? Are they fully utilized? Do you need more staff, less staff, or different staff? Are your facilities adequate? Finances adequate? What are your major strengths? Weaknesses?

Step 3. Define the business climate in your industry. (How is the weather and what is the forecast?) Do you expect this situation to improve or worsen during the next year? Five years? How does it affect your company?

Step 4. Determine your major goals and objectives. (Where are you going? Cross country or nearest airfield?) Do you want to maintain your current size? Grow? Why? Do you want more profit? Why more profit? New equipment? Investment? Do you want to broaden or narrow the scope of operations?

Step 5. Determine the strategies necessary to achieve those goals. (What route are you taking?) Do you need to hire staff? How will you recruit? New facilities? Where? What kind? What will they cost? Do you need more capital?

Step 6. Set up short- and long-range schedules for achieving your stated goals. (How long will it take to get there?) What tasks need to be accomplished during the next six months? Next year? Next five years?

Step 7. Assign staff responsibilities for each activity in the plan (if you have a crew). What are the duties of your staff? Who will check to be sure they are carried out? What is the reporting process? How often?

Step 8. Develop a realistic budget to support each objective. (How do you plan to pay for the trip?) What are your monthly expenses? What is your monthly revenue? Can you make a profit? How long will it take you to get paid by your customers? Can you financially support your plans? Do you need borrowing capability? Loans? Will you need additional capital?

Step 9. Establish target dates for review and updating of plans. (What do your instruments tell you about this flight?) Is it working? Why or why not? What do you need to change? Is there money left to do it? Was the money spent in a cost-effective manner? What are the results to date?

Keep in mind that plans are meant to be carried out, not simply read, filed, and forgotten. The text is less important than the managerial information you have developed as a result of effective planning and the action taken. Incomplete planning can cause serious problems.

> *Example*: In one state a question recently arose about private rehabilitation providers being regulated as employment agencies. This additional regulation would present considerable problems for the private providers within the state from a cost standpoint. Such a change would require a change in the way they do business in order to meet state requirements under this law. Also, the change would allow dual regulation on many issues by two state agencies. Legislation was introduced to exempt the private rehabilitation organizations from this law. Unfortunately, the private providers did not have a lobbyist work with them to be sure this legislation came to the attention of their legislators. No cohesive effort was made on the part of any particular provider or group of providers to see that this legislation was called to the attention of the legislators. The legislation was not enacted. Therefore, at this time the state is in the process of bringing the private rehabilitation providers under the employment agency provisions of the law. This is going to be costly and time-consuming to all of the providers within the state. No plan was developed by either the private providers as individuals or by their professional organizations to deal with this anticipated problem.

In the planning process these individuals got only to Step 2, that of identifying and evaluating the problem. However, they did not set a goal, develop strategies, schedules, and responsibilities, or budgets to deal with this problem. Therefore, nothing happened to prevent the problem. Now they are all facing a crisis.

Summary

Planning is essential for effective business management. A business plan includes goals and objectives, strategies to accomplish the goals, and a determination of the resources needed. Planning is a continual process based on feedback, evaluation of results, and revision of the plan based on new information. The development and continual refinement of your business plan is essential if you are to achieve your goals.

Appendix: Recommended Reading

Cohen, W. A., & Reddick, M. E. *Successful marketing for small businesses.* New York: AMACOM, 1981.

Hopkins, D. S. *The marketing plan.* New York: The Conference Board, 1981.

Seiler, G. R. *Control – The key to successful business planning.* New York: AMACOM, 1981.

Webb, S. G. *Marketing & strategic planning for professional service firms.* New York: AMACOM, 1982.

Wortman, L. A. *Successful small business management.* New York: AMACOM, 1976.

13 Being an Ethical Professional in Private Sector Rehabilitation

Lewis J. Taylor

Introduction

The emergence of the profession of rehabilitation, especially its private sector, has created numerous ethical dilemmas for its practitioners. By its very nature as a social system designed to help individuals reach their own goals, rehabilitation has an inherent conflict that creates some of these dilemmas. The purpose of this chapter is to help the rehabilitation professional conceptualize and resolve ethical dilemmas peculiar to rehabilitation in the private sector. Of course, the basic concepts involved are applicable to all rehabilitation settings. After a discussion of philosophical foundations, professional ethics, and their interrelationship, the ethics codes especially relevant to private sector rehabilitationists will be identified. Several characteristics of private sector rehabilitation that produce ethical dilemmas will then be described. Subsequently, a number of ethical dilemmas will be presented and resolved by reference to rehabilitation's philosophical foundations and ethical codes. By this means, the author hopes to illustrate for the reader a method for resolving ethical dilemmas by using rehabilitation's philosophical foundations and existing ethical codes and statements. The reader may not agree with the author's solutions to the ethical problems presented in this chapter, but he or she will be able to go to the relevant philosophical and ethical resources to look for the solutions just as the author has. While the method used here is sound, the resources it employs are admittedly imperfect. As practitioners apply current ethical statements to real life problems in the private sector, they will find that improvements can be made, and they will make them. It is not an objective of this chapter to criticize the current ethical statements, but simply to use them, imperfect as they may be, to help private sector practitioners resolve ethical dilemmas as they find them now.

The Problem

The application of theory to practice raises thorny ethical problems in any field. The medical field is currently grappling with the dilemma created by the availability of medical technology that can artificially prolong life. On the one hand, the physician has a responsibility to prevent the patient from dying. On the other hand, futile efforts can bankrupt a family. What is one to do? It is safe to say that there is not yet a consensus in the medical profession or in our society on this question.

Not all ethical dilemmas are so dramatic, but they can be troublesome in similar ways. The private sector rehabilitation professional today is often asking "What am I to do?" when confronting the ethical dilemmas peculiar to this field. How does one resolve, for instance, the problem created by the client's demand for a rehabilitation plan that would "actualize his potential" when the sponsor of that plan (such as an insurance company) refuses to pay for it? How does the rehabilitation professional meet the ethical requirement of confidentiality when scores of people (e.g., attorneys, insurance workers, and government personnel) have full access to the client's file? How does one properly integrate the "profit motive" and the "service motive" in private practice to avoid exploiting clients or others in the effort to put bread and butter on the table? In short, how does the professional, providing rehabilitation services on a private fee-for-service basis practice ethically? This chapter will attempt to answer these questions.

Several authors have addressed the unique characteristics that create ethical dilemmas in private sector rehabilitation and have discussed the need for ethics specifically suited to the private sector practitioner. A brief review of this literature follows.

A Brief Review of the Literature

Since the sudden development of private sector rehabilitation in the mid-seventies, there has been considerable discussion in the literature about ethical problems related to this area of the rehabilitation profession. Several authors have described some of the unique characteristics of private sector rehabilitation, characteristics that have produced some uncertainty about ethical behavior among its practitioners. Only a few authors have made any attempt to provide specific ethical guidance to the private sector professional.

Scher (1979) has pointedly noted the need for ethical standards in private sector rehabilitation, standards which would specifically address problems unique to this field. He states that the need for special ethical standards is due to the diversity of the backgrounds of private practitioners, some of whom, he asserts, are unqualified. An ethical standard, Scher argues, would enable the profession to police itself. The National Association of Rehabilitation Professionals in the Private Sector (NARPPS) can, Scher suggests, provide a forum for the examination of ethical issues, among others.

The growing consumer movement is making it evermore important for all professional groups to set ethical standards and to police themselves. Glaser (1981) notes that review and redefinition of ethical practices are under way in all professions as professional activity is coming under increasing government control and public scrutiny. According to Glaser, a consulting psychologist, every consulting professional must build a personal professional code of ethics by starting with the ethical standards of his own professional group. This for Glaser would be the ethics of the American Psychological Association. This is apt advice for rehabilitation with its diverse array of practitioners. Like the consultant, the rehabilitationist should look to his own professional group (e.g., occupational therapy, vocational evaluation, rehabilitation counseling, etc.) for an ethical starting place. Glaser also, like McMahon (1979), urges the teaching of ethics in the graduate schools. Glaser adds that business organizations should involve their employees, as some have, in developing their own sets of rules of conduct. In some cases, Glaser notes, this effort has been rewarded by reductions in union-management grievances and absenteeism and increases in overall job satisfaction.

Ross (1979) and Welch (1979), respectively, note the importance of ethical standards. According to Ross, if a private rehabilitation program does not operate ethically, it will not, in the long run, be able to compete with those that do. Similarly, Welch states that it "would seem imperative that private-for-profit vendors not compromise their rehabilitation efforts in favor of the insurance industry . . . the private-for-profit rehabilitation professional must guard against vulnerability to this charge" (1979, p. 31).

Concern for ethics is not limited to the academicians and leaders in the field. In a training needs survey by Lynch and Martin (1982), private sector rehabilitation counselors indicated that rehabilitation counseling philosophy and professional ethics are important training topics. Of 41 topics, only five were considered more important than professional ethics. While rehabilitation counseling philosophy was rated "important" by responding counselors, 32 topics were rated as being more important. Counselors are apparently more concerned with practical ethical problems than with the underlying philosophical basis of ethics.

Several writers have suggested reasons for the special importance of ethics in private sector rehabilitation. McMahon (1979) notes the lack of other controls in the free enterprise system, the vested interests of the several parties to each case, and the variety of practitioners. Lewin, Ramseur, and Sink (1979) note the skepticism the public sector has of the private sector due to the latter's profit orientation. They argue, however, that many private practitioners value the ethical standards learned in their training and believe that profits can be earned ethically. Ultimately, these authors conclude, the opportunity for the rehabilitation professional to provide valuable human services for which private industry is willing to pay can only be good for the profession. Deneen and Hessellund (1981) argue that "third party involvement," by the insurance company, for example, is the private sector characteristic that creates most of its ethical dilemmas. The authors claim that the traditional ethics statements of groups like the National Rehabilitation Counseling Association fail to address this third party issue and thus are of little help to the private practitioner.

Deneen and Hessellund (1981) go further than most other writers in offering specific guidance for counselors in handling private sector ethical problems involving relationships with clients and referral sources, confidentiality, billing, and marketing. Sanchez, et al. (1981) also offer concrete ethical guidance to practitioners regarding the "ethical responsibility to establish and maintain adequate relationships with all parties involved in the vocational rehabilitation process" (p. 175). The authors identify several benefits that come from having knowledge of and respect for each party's rights, being objective and competent in interaction with others, having adequate documentation of rehabilitation services, and being available to all parties.

This brief review of the literature suggests that private sector practitioners and observers agree that ethics are important. Some believe that special ethics statements are necessary. Overall, there seems to be more interest in ethical rules than in the philosophical foundations that should underlie those rules. The opinion of this author is that ethics statements already in circulation provide adequate guidance as long as they are used in the context of the philosophical foundations of rehabilitation (see Taylor, 1980). As Glaser (1981) has suggested to consulting psychologists, rehabilitationists would benefit from reexamining their respective professional standards and ethics to find a basis for the development of personal ethical rules to guide their behavior in the private sector.

The remainder of this chapter will show the relationship between philosophical foundations and ethics and will show the reader how to use existing ethics statements to solve dilemmas peculiar to private sector rehabilitation.

Philosophical Foundations and Professional Ethics

The philosophical foundations of a field of study or endeavor are composed of the basic beliefs, assumptions, principles, and values that, according to Beatrice Wright (1972), "when commonly shared give a direction or stamp to the field" (p. 38). A professional ethics is an explicit set of values governing the professional behavior of an individual who offers professional service. A profession's ethics should be derived from its philosophical foundations.

Philosophical foundations may or may not be clearly stated, but they are always present. The same may be said for ethics. The human being has beliefs, assumptions, principles, values, and rules of conduct whether or not he or she recognizes them and can define them. The person ordinarily acts consistently. This is why the concept of personality can be postulated. This consistent behavior is an observable consequence of an underlying, invisible, philosophical foundation. Just as the walls of a house are visible extensions of its foundation, professional ethics, as rules of behavior, are extensions of philosophical foundations.

In any profession, it is desirable for its practitioners to behave consistently and positively. With positive and consistent professional behavior come better service for the client and more prosperity for the profession. Professional groups have, then, written codes of ethics to which all members of the group are expected to subscribe. These ethics statements are derived from philosophical foundations which may or may not have been clearly stated. In the field of rehabilitation, for instance, while there are statements of professional ethics, there is no thorough, clear published description of its philosophical foundations (Taylor, 1980). This is not to say, of course, that it has none. In the next section, the philosophical foundations of rehabilitation will be presented.

The Philosophical Foundations of Rehabilitation

In the rehabilitation literature, there are many references to the philosophy of rehabilitation and even a few relatively formal statements of values, objectives, and beliefs (American Psychological Association, 1972; Wright, 1972). However, in these statements there is no elaboration of the philosophical foundation that would support these ideas (Taylor, 1980).

Several writers have noted and complained about this oversight. Keith (1969) has written that physical rehabilitation "does not currently have such a philosophy" (p. 170). Dellario (1978) has complained that rehabilitation research has been plagued by incoherence stemming from the lack of a common rehabilitation research perspective that a clearly stated philosophical foundation could provide. In a recent (and rare) discussion of philosophy and ethics in rehabilitation counseling, Bozarth (1981) notes that the "lack of specific statements . . . may be detrimental to the future of rehabilitation counseling as a profession" (p. 60). Bozarth goes on to discuss the philosophical presuppositions of rehabilitation counseling and offers several propositions for the development of a philosophical framework (or foundation) for the profession.

In an effort to identify the philosophical principles that influence rehabilitation practice, Taylor (1980) conducted an analysis of the writing of rehabilitationists of three different orientations: psychoanalytic, somato-psychological, and behavioral. On the basis of this analysis, several major principles were identified, principles that could provide the blocks for the building of a philosophical foundation for rehabilitation. The principles are

1. The goal of rehabilitation is adjustment between the disabled person and the environment.
2. The rehabilitationist defines adjustment as the person's creative adaptation of his or her capabilities to the environment's requirements and opportunities.
3. The person has value as an individual.
4. The person is a whole, a living synthesis, and thus his or her personality cannot be understood in terms of a particular disability.
5. The person is ultimately a conscious self.
6. The person interacts with the environment actively, purposefully, and in a direction consistent with his perceptions of himself and the environment.
7. The person is responsible for his or her behavior.
8. The person knows what is good for himself or herself.
9. The individual person is a unique being and cannot be understood simply in terms of statistical averages or social mores.
10. Rehabilitation stresses assets and well-behavior over deficits and sick-behavior.
11. The rehabilitationist, whether studying interpersonal relations, intrapersonal dynamics, or behavior change, always begins the study with empathy for the person's private point of view.
12. Rehabilitation recognizes the deficiencies in professional knowledge and therefore relies on comanagement of the rehabilitation process by the professional and the client.
13. Caring for the client by the rehabilitation professional is important for rehabilitation success.
14. The rehabilitationist conducts research on the basis of faith in analysis and operational definitions and with regard for each of the principles and practices described above.
15. Rehabilitation stresses the significance of environmental factors in aggravating or ameliorating the handicapping effects of disability and, therefore, argues for an ethic of social responsibility to eliminate environmental barriers to adjustment.

In the Taylor study these principles were compared to the major tenets of the "humanistic-existential" orientation (or "Third Force") in psychology, and it was concluded that they are congruent. He recommended that the humanistic-existential orientation be used as the basis for the development of a firm and broad foundation for rehabilitation (Taylor, 1980).

Taking a different approach, Bozarth (1981) identified several propositions that are compatible with the principles listed above. These are

1. All individuals possess human dignity and worth regardless of their disability or limitations.
2. Disabled individuals can become self-sufficient and can contribute to society.
3. Productive activity, employment, and/or maximum vocational independence are important psychological benefits to individuals.
4. Individuals' participation and determination of their own plans and destinies are essential elements in rehabilitation.
5. Diagnostic techniques, therapeutic intervention, environmental alterations, and activation of services for clients can be combined to produce effective results (p. 67–69).

The clear congruence of Bozarth's "propositions" and Taylor's "principles" is further evidence of the presence of sufficiently consistent ideas with which to build an explicit philosophical foundation for rehabilitation. In the next section, the subject of professional ethics is addressed with primary attention to the major current ethics statements relevant to the rehabilitation profession.

The Professional Ethics of Rehabilitation

A professional code of ethics is written to set rules of behavior to insure that the interests of the profession and its client are well served. Shertzer and Stone (Bozarth, 1981) have described the major purposes of an ethical code as follows:

1. Provides a position on standards of practice to assist each member of the profession in deciding what he should do when situations of conflict arise in his work;
2. Helps clarify the counselor's responsibility to the client and protects the client from the counselor's violation of, or his failure to fulfill, these responsibilities;
3. Gives the profession some assurance that the practices of members will not be detrimental to its general functions and purposes;

4. Gives society some guarantee that the services of the counselor will demonstrate a sensible regard for the social codes and moral expectations of the community in which he works;
5. Offers the counselor himself some grounds for safeguarding his own privacy and integrity (p. 71).

Three codes of ethics have special relevance here. The first, published by the National Rehabilitation Counseling Association (NRCA) in 1972 was designed for use by all rehabilitation counselors. Of course, in 1972 almost all counselors worked in public or private nonprofit settings, so some issues peculiar to the private-for-profit sector are not explicitly treated in the NRCA code. The second was published by the National Association of Rehabilitation Professionals in the Private Sector (NARPPS) in 1981. Since NARPPS is composed of rehabilitation professionals who practice in the private-for-profit sector, its Standards and Ethics primarily addresses issues peculiar to this area. The third is the Code of Ethics published by the Vocational Evaluation and Work Adjustment Association (VEWAA) (1971).

Taken together, the NRCA, NARPPS, and VEWAA statements provide the private sector rehabilitation professional (including counselors, evaluators, and others) with a set of guidelines for ethical professional practice. These guidelines are imperfect to be sure, but they are helpful, nevertheless. Furthermore, if the counselor understands and uses these guidelines *within the context of the philosophical foundations of rehabilitation* described above, the usefulness and validity of the ethics guidelines are improved.[1]

The reader should obtain copies of these ethical codes and statements. The NARPPS Standards and Ethics is contained here as an appendix because of its particular interest to the private practitioner. These ethics will be used throughout the rest of this chapter to demonstrate how we may resolve ethical dilemmas in private sector rehabilitation.

Causes of Ethical Dilemmas in Private Sector

There are several characteristics of the private sector that necessarily produce ethical dilemmas for the practitioner because of the way these characteristics interact with the philosophical foundations and ethics of rehabilitation. It is important to keep in mind the distinction implied here.

[1]Codes of ethics of other related professional groups such as those published by the American Psychological Association (APA, 1977) and the American Personnel and Guidance Association (APGA, 1976) can also help the rehabilitation practitioner in certain situations. However, these will not be used in this discussion for the sake of simplicity.

Rehabilitation and the private sector are not the same thing. The private sector is simply an "arena" in which rehabilitation can be practiced. The public sector is another arena. The way rehabilitation is practiced will differ from arena to arena just as baseball or football tactics vary from field to field. Nevertheless, it is rehabilitation that is practiced, just as it is baseball that is played regardless of the size and shape of the ballpark. Rehabilitation is a process that can be employed in a variety of settings to meet a variety of challenges. The private sector practitioner is demonstrating this every day. By reference to the ground rules provided by ethics and philosophical foundations, rehabilitation can be practiced "fair and square" in any setting.

The Profit Motive

An important characteristic of the private sector is the profit motive. That is, the rehabilitation professional is not restricted to a salary schedule but is able to increase his or her income by working efficiently and hard. For the professional in the private sector, the paycheck may not be something that can be taken for granted. For the rehabilitationist in private practice, income is completely dependent on his or her own efforts. There is potential in this condition for conflict between the professional's need for income and his or her provision of services. At the worst, the profit motive can encourage the provision of rehabilitation services that are not in the client's interest. At the best, the professional can be influenced by the profit motive to do the best job possible. The direction one takes depends upon many factors, including how he or she understands and uses the philosophical foundations and ethics of rehabilitation.

Competition

The same may be said for other characteristics of the private sector such as competition. Competition between practitioners in a given geographic area for a finite number of case referrals presents them with choices that can be better made by reference to professional ethics. Rehabilitation professionals are finding themselves in competition with each other not only in the marketplace but in the courtroom. Rehabilitation services (vocational evaluation, for instance) are increasingly being used by attorneys to support their cases. Rehabilitation professionals can find themselves testifying on either side of the legal arguments. These are relatively new experiences for rehabilitation practitioners, and there should be little wonder that many feel unsure about handling these challenges.

Litigation

Many of the areas that provide opportunities for rehabilitation practitioners in the private sector are fraught with legal factors. Workers' compensation is a good example. Even though the various state workers' compensation systems are devised to be administrative rather than judicial systems, attorneys are nevertheless involved. Many workers' compensation claimants believe they need attorneys to help them obtain their benefits from the system. Thus, the rehabilitation counselor is faced with practical problems as well as ethical dilemmas not present when he or she deals simply and directly with the client in the private nonprofit setting.

Vested Interests

In the workers' compensation system as well as other insurance and government systems, the rehabilitation counselor (and often the client) is continually buffeted by often contradictory vested interests. The state wants to protect the rights of the individual and increase tax receipts. The employer or the insurance carrier wants to minimize the cost of the case and close it successfully. The client's (claimant's) attorney believes it is best to maximize his client's disability rating. The counselor believes it is best to maximize the client's ability. The client is torn between getting all he or she can from "the system" and getting back to work to provide for the family. Obviously, all these pressures will be felt by the counselor trying to develop a rehabilitation plan or the vocational evaluator trying to conduct a work evaluation. How these pressures are handled will influence the quality of service the client receives in the short run, and, in the long run, it will affect the development of rehabilitation as a profession.

Rehabilitation Goals

One characteristic of the private sector that appears to be different from the public or private nonprofit sector is that the goal of the rehabilitation effort is established by the benefit system (such as Social Security or workers' compensation) rather than the rehabilitationist or the client. Traditionally, the goal of rehabilitation has been to fulfill the client's potential for work or independent living. In the benefit systems within which private practitioners often work, the goal may be simply to return the client to suitable gainful employment as soon as practicable. Realization of vocational potential may be regarded as an unaffordable luxury in these systems. The counselor who has been trained to work toward traditional goals may experience an ethical dilemma when told to simply "get the client back to work."

Diversity of Practitioners

There is a great diversity of background and training of practitioners in the private sector (Matkin, 1981). This diversity adds to the potential for ethical dilemmas in the field. In the California workers' compensation system, for example (Division of Industrial Accidents, 1979), anyone who is "qualified" can work with a disabled person to develop a rehabilitation plan. Experience and academic qualifications are only vaguely spelled out. This situation is not unique to California. Across the country, people with academic credentials from the high-school diploma to the Ph.D. degree are providing rehabilitation services for a fee. This, combined with the variety of professional types in rehabilitation (such as nurses, counselors, evaluators, occupational therapists, psychologists, and job developers, to name some) provides an environment for ethical dilemmas to arise. Can all these people agree on the nature of advocacy for the disabled, or the importance of confidentiality, or the need for vocational evaluation, or work adjustment or job placement? An adequate understanding of the philosophical bases and professional ethics can provide a basis for effective communication between practitioners of diverse backgrounds.

The "Outlaw Image"

Many private sector rehabilitation practitioners have felt like "outlaws" from their profession. Separation of the rehabilitation profession into nonprofit and for-profit sectors has produced real anxiety and stress in some practitioners. Practitioners in the traditional settings have sometimes accused private sector practitioners of being less than professional. Private sector rehabilitation professionals sometimes believe their "bad press." Indeed, there are aspects of private sector rehabilitation that can encourage unprofessional behavior. But, as noted above, rehabilitation is rehabilitation. It is synonymous neither with the state-federal system nor with the workers' compensation system nor with Goodwill Industries. Supported by a strong philosophical foundation and armed with an adequate code of ethics, the rehabilitation practitioner can practice ethically in any setting.

Ethical Dilemmas: Illustrated and Resolved

Most of the rest of this chapter will be devoted to illustrating some of the ethical dilemmas in private sector rehabilitation and suggesting solutions to these dilemmas. In this way, the foregoing generalizations can be made concrete. In each of the following examples, this format will be repeated: the dilemma will be illustrated, the relevant ethical and or philosophical statement will be quoted, and a solution to the dilemma will be suggested. The author does not profess to be an ethical judge for the profession. The reader may disagree with the solution or even doubt the existence of the dilemma. This chapter will have met its objective if the reader is stimulated to think about his or her own ethical dilemmas and how they might be solved.

Client's Demands versus Others' Expectations

The rehabilitation counselor will undoubtedly face a client one day whose vocational goals conflict with those of the institutions prepared to pay for the necessary services. In some cases, the client is unrealistic in his goal setting. In other cases, the client is being unnecessarily and perhaps unfairly restricted in his goal setting by the "holders of the purse." At other times, both the client's goals and others' expectations are equally unreasonable. It is the counselor who is expected to resolve these conflicts. But how? One cannot simply take the client's side or the "system's" side. There are ethical proscriptions against both courses of action (NRCA, 1972). By referring to the philosophical statement given above that "the goal of rehabilitation is adjustment between the disabled person and his environment" (Taylor, 1980, p. 110), we find a clue. That is, the solution will require flexibility and adaptation to circumstances to make the adjustment. In the NRCA Ethical Standards, we find in Section VIII, B, that if "the counselor cannot concur in the rehabilitation plan for a client referred to him he will resolve the differences between the plan and what he believes should be done" (1972, p. 355). So here we find clear guidance about what to do. The counselor will not simply forge a compromise between the client and the system, instead he or she will compare the unacceptable plan, whether it is the client's or the insurance carrier's, to what *should be done* according to rehabilitation's standards of practice and the system's rules and regulations.

Let us see how these ideas might apply to a real-life situation. Take the case of a bright, 20-year-old paraplegic whose personal rehabilitation plan to complete the third and fourth years of a B.A. degree program already underway is turned down by the self-insured employer as being too long and expensive. The counselor could simply negotiate a compromise between the client and the employer—say, financial support for the junior year but not for the senior year. This course of action, however, sidesteps the rehabilitation problem. The counselor, following the philosophical principle and ethical statement quoted above, could analyze the plan and evaluate it in the light of the client's characteristics and labor market factors. Then, with reference to the rules and regulations of the applicable benefit system, the counselor could systematically determine the appropriateness of the student's program. The point here is that, to be ethical, the counselor must practice rehabilitation, not mere negotiation and compromise.

In the following paragraphs other ethical dilemmas will be presented and resolved.

The Profit versus the Service Orientation

Rehabilitation is a human service based on respect and caring for the individual. The private sector rehabilitationist is not only providing a human service but is also pursuing a profit. What is the vocational evaluator to do when confronted by a brain-damaged client referred for vocational evaluation when the evaluator has never worked with a brain-damaged client before and is essentially unfamiliar with the psychological, social, and physical implications of this disability? The profit motive might push the evaluator to accept the referral and just try to do the best he can. The service orientation would lead the evaluator to refer the client on to someone more familiar with the particular disability.

Both the VEWAA and the NARPPS ethics statements address this situation in several ways. This abundance of attention is necessary as this dilemma is related to many of the ethical dilemmas faced in private sector rehabilitation. The VEWAA Code of Ethics addresses this issue in two of its principles, "Professional Competence" and "Interprofessional Relationships." Specifically, the VEWAA Code insists that the evaluator "should be fully cognizant of the level and nature of his professional competence and recognize that in attempting to perform beyond his levels and areas of competency, he may endanger the welfare of those he serves" (1971, p. 26). With regard to interprofessional relationships, the code advises the evaluator to "refer to, and seek the services of, those professionally qualified to deal with problems or situations outside of his province" (1971, p. 27).

The NARPPS Standards and Ethics (1981) states that the "member shall render only those services that the member is competent and qualified to perform." Furthermore, the NARPPS "member has an obligation to withdraw from a professional relationship if it is believed that the participation will result in the violation of the ethical standards of his/her discipline." Money can be lost by such caution, but the intent of these ethical statements is clear. The evaluator in our example may be disappointed by the loss of this client, but he should not be uncertain about the ethical course of action. Of course, the philosophical principle that caring for the client is important for rehabilitation success is relevant here, too (Taylor, 1980).

Confidentiality

In the traditional rehabilitation service delivery system, client confidentiality is generally tightly guarded. Release of records or information about the client generally requires the completion of medical or professional release forms by the client. In some nontraditional rehabilitation benefit systems, however, a free flow of client information and records among interested parties is commonplace. In some workers' compensation systems, for example, the client is presumed to have given up a large measure of his right to privacy by accepting the benefits offered. In California, workers' compensation medical records are routinely and legally passed from physician to insurance carrier to employer to attorney to the state's rehabilitation bureau and so on without the use of medical release forms. The public nature of the client's file can leave the concerned rehabilitation professional unsure of his or her responsibilities in this ethical area.

The NRCA and NARPPS statements again provide guidance. Section VIII, E, of the NRCA statement emphasizes the counselor's responsibility to protect "information confidentiality" but adds that "information necessary for the cooperating agencies to be effective in serving the client will be promptly supplied by the referring counselor" (NRCA, 1972, p. 355). But, the information "will be limited to that which is necessary to effect delivery of service" (NRCA, 1972, p. 356). The NARPPS statement (1981) suggests that the way to handle the public nature of the benefit system is to "make certain that the client is aware from the outset, that the delivery of services is being observed by a third party." The VEWAA code likewise advises that clients be made aware in advance of administrative and legal limits of confidentiality (1971). The rehabilitationist in the private sector then can take heart that, at least according to the NRCA, it is ethical to share information as necessary about the client with cooperating agencies such as the insurance carrier. But he should take note that this should be done only after telling the client about the limits of confidentiality in the given benefit system. (The reader should refer to the NRCA Ethical Standards and the VEWAA Codes of Ethics for fuller elaboration of ethical guidelines for confidentiality.)

Evaluation versus Treatment

The benefit systems within which many private sector rehabilitationists work (such as workers' compensation and Social Security) emphasize evaluation over treatment. A dilemma for the private sector counselor lies in his or her recognition of a need for some intervention (such as psychological counseling or work adjustment services) for a client who is not eligible for such services according to system rules and regulations or conventions. In some systems, clients may be judged by work evaluators to be "unfeasible" candidates for rehabilitation services for physical or psychological reasons. Their rehabilitation benefits are then suspended, and they are on their own to correct the problems which created the "unfeasibility." Many rehabilitationists would feel frustrated by this situation, not being able to refer for or to provide therapeutic interventions such as work adjustment or psychological counseling. This situation not only frustrates the counselor but also raises a serious question of ethical responsibility.

Perhaps because this problem has become especially apparent with the development of private sector rehabilitation, the NARPPS statement gives more explicit guidance in this dilemma than the NRCA statement. The NRCA statement merely calls on the counselor to "protect the client's welfare and . . . assist the client toward his goals" (1972, p. 340). The NARPPS statement (1981) indicates that the "role of the NARPPS member as an advocate is to protect and promote the welfare of disabled persons to maximize control over circumstances that interfere with their obtaining vocational independence." On the other hand, the NARPPS "member shall refuse to participate in practices which are inconsistent with the standards established by regulatory bodies regarding the delivery of services to clients." The implied instruction to the rehabilitationist here would seem to be to do everything he or she can do, within the parameters of the relevant rehabilitation benefit system, to remove the rehabilitation barriers the client faces. When the client needs services the system is not equipped or prepared to provide, the counselor should advise the client on how to obtain these services elsewhere. For example, a disabled worker experiencing marital conflict that interferes with the rehabilitation effort might be referred to a community family counseling center, through the benefit system if it allows, or around it if it does not. Ultimately, of course, it is not the rehabilitationist's duty to do everything for the client. A review of basic rehabilitation principles (Taylor, 1980) shows the emphasis rehabilitation places on developing the abilities and independence of the client.

Competition among Rehabilitation Professionals

There are two common arenas in which rehabilitation professionals find themselves in direct competition—the marketplace and the courtroom. Most rehabilitationists are unfamiliar with both settings and their demands and are thus often unaware of how to handle the ethical dilemmas they pose. Competition in the marketplace may be rewarding, but it is very risky. The rehabilitationist either wins in this competition or he goes out of business. Most often the competition is for case referrals which, of course, result eventually in income. One dilemma this competition presents is that described earlier as "profit motive versus service orientation." Another is the temptation to criticize one's colleagues in the effort to attract referrals to one's own practice. Many new private sector rehabilitationists have succumbed to this temptation and then felt a little queasy afterward, and with good reason. Both the NRCA and the NARPPS statements are quite clear about the ethical implications of this kind of competitive behavior.

In the NRCA statement, Section IV, C, states that the "counselor will not disseminate information about his colleagues that would tend to erode their professional status or effectiveness" (1972, p. 351). The NARPPS statement (1981) provides several ethical guidelines regarding business practices. In particular, "members will not misrepresent themselves, their duties or their credentials." Nor will they engage in "any discussion, comments, or criticism directed toward a fellow Professional Rehabilitation Practitioner or organization [that is not] positive/constructive." Of course, it is only the naive professional who sells his or her services by criticizing the competition. Describing one's own positive characteristics is far more effective.

Competition in the courtroom is even more direct. Here one rehabilitationist may take the stand after another, confront the same facts, and render a different conclusion. Can this be ethical? Is not one of them lying, or at least distorting the truth a little? Not necessarily. Rehabilitation is part of the behavioral sciences and thus is as much art as science. That is, the variables are numerous and complex, and many are not well understood. There is much room for disagreement between experts in assessing vocational handicap which is the issue about which most rehabilitationists are called to testify. Our two experts might make different starting assumptions about the facts or issues in the case and thus reach different conclusions.

For example, a recent case involved a machinist who had suffered skin irritation from contact with the cutting oils common to his trade. At issue was the degree to which the worker was vocationally handicapped. Both vocational evaluators measured this handicap by counting the number of jobs the worker was unable to do because of the skin irritation. One evaluator counted only those jobs that required contact with cutting oils while the other evaluator counted all jobs that required contact with *any* potentially irritating materials *and* those jobs the worker could do by virtue of his profile of aptitudes. Of course, the first evaluator assessed a lesser degree of disability than the second. Neither assessment was unethical. Each assessment had a sound rationale. They were both based on facts, and both evaluators were qualified by training and experience to render their opinions. Competence and objectivity are the primary benchmarks for ethical testimony, according to the NARPPS statement (1981).

Competition in private sector rehabilitation has already resulted in real improvements in services, especially in the area of evaluation. However, if private sector rehabilitation is to develop as a profession and not merely an industry, its competitive practices must be those of a profession.

The Exploitation of the System by the Client

Rehabilitationists are by training prepared to deal with exploitation of the client by the system. But what of exploitation of the system by the client? The financial rewards of disability are great in some systems (such as the federal longshoremen's and harbor workers' program). The natural motivation of most of us to work can be diverted by the financial disincentives found in most benefit systems. Several of Taylor's principles (1980) remind us that the client acts consciously, actively, and purposefully on the basis of what he or she perceives to be self-interest. Some clients are motivated to participate in rehabilitation services because of the related cash benefits but are reluctant to complete the rehabilitation process with job placement because the new job brings the termination of those cash benefits. The counselor or evaluator whose client is apparently faking or exaggerating symptoms or is dragging his feet in the vocational exploration process can face an ethical dilemma; that is, to tell or not to tell. Curiously, the NARPPS statement is silent on this issue. The NRCA statement is not: "The counselor will take action to correct the situation where the client is improperly exploiting the agencies involved in the client's rehabilitation" (NRCA, 1972, p. 355).

In the case of the client who seems to be purposefully prolonging the vocational exploration process in order to collect cash benefits, the counselor will act ethically by confronting him with his behavior. If this fails to bring a redirection of the client's motivation, then the counselor would arrange for a conference between all the parties to the case in order to discuss the client's behavior and its implications for rehabilitation. It is a well-accepted rehabilitation principle that rehabilitation is a joint effort between the client and the counselor (Taylor, 1980). It cannot effectively proceed without honest confrontation and communication.

Changing Jobs and Taking Cases

Counselor-employees who chose to move from one rehabilitation service firm to another face an ethical dilemma. So do those who decide to leave their firm to begin a private practice or a company of their own. This dilemma is whether or not to take cases the counselor is working on to the new place of employment. Recruiters might encourage the counselor to take cases to the new job. The counselor himself would be tempted to do so, especially if beginning a private practice where just a few cases more or less can bring success or failure.

In its only specific reference to this dilemma, the NARPPS statement (1981) insists that no "Professional Rehabilitation Practitioner or organization shall effectuate or participate in the wrongful removal of professional rehabilitation files or other materials upon the initiation of new employment." According to the NRCA ethics, when the counselor decides to leave his position he "will give his employer timely and adequate advance notice and will leave his work in such condition that the successor can continue effective service to the clients" (1972, p. 354). The implication, though not directly stated, is that the client is primarily the client of the agency and secondarily the client of the counselor-employee. But what if the counselor strongly believes that it is in the best interest of the client to continue the counselor-client relationship at the new place of employment? Traditionally, counselors have resolved this dilemma by discussing the case with the agency management and other parties to the case to explain why the case should remain with the counselor. With the agreement of all parties, the counselor-client relationship would then continue. In this way, the ethical imperatives for the counselor to care for and work for the welfare of the client on the one hand, and to "be loyal to the agency that employs him" (NRCA, 1972, p. 353) on the other hand, can both be satisfied.

Conclusion

These examples of ethical dilemmas in private sector rehabilitation illustrate two important points. First, ethical dilemmas are practical matters, not just philosophical ones. It really matters to the client whether he will receive work adjustment services to facilitate his return to work. It really matters to the counselor whether or not he is able to take cases with him when he leaves the agency for private practice. Second, ethical dilemmas have no easy answers. The foregoing discussion has necessarily been simplistic. For example, the dilemma of whether or not the rehabilitationist should serve as the client's advocate in private sector rehabilitation, a dilemma which has been addressed only indirectly here, is one which cannot be resolved by reference to sentences in any code of ethics. Rather, the practitioner must be familiar with all relevant ethical statements as well as the philosophical foundations of rehabilitation in order to forge an ethical decision by the synthesis of a variety of sometimes contradictory ideas. In this way then, the practitioner might come to the conclusion that his primary obligation to champion the welfare of the client should be tempered by the understanding that the client is responsible for his own behavior and by a concern for the welfare of the society-at-large.

Rehabilitation is still an emerging profession (Brubaker, 1981). Neither its philosophical foundations nor its ethical statements are thoroughly developed. While rehabilitation principles are commonly referred to in the literature, the philosophical foundations from which they are derived have not yet been made explicit in a formal and systematic way. While various organizations have published ethics relevant to private sector rehabilitationists, these ethics leave many issues unanswered or incompletely addressed. Nevertheless, the efforts that have been made to explicate philosophical foundations and to write ethical codes are giant steps in the right direction. The concern expressed every day by rehabilitation professionals grappling with real life ethical problems will, it is hoped, stimulate further thoughtful work in this area.

In the meantime, the resources we already have should be used by rehabilitation professionals—counselor-employees and private practitioners alike—to develop a greater awareness of ethical dilemmas and to provide a stronger basis for ethical decision making. Rehabilitation service firms and university graduate programs have a special responsibility. Counseling staffs and graduate classes should be provided with explicit statements of philosophical foundations and ethics by supervisors and professors who demonstrate by their own work behavior that they care about these issues. The various certification and accreditation programs of rehabilitation disciplines should be supported and further developed. Their importance in encouraging ethical professional behavior is great.

Finally, we rehabilitation professionals should confront each other regularly on matters of ethical concern. By doing this, as well as by actively using relevant ethical codes to solve ethical problems, we will all feel better, knowing that we are doing the best we can to meet the ethical responsibilities of our professional lives.

Appendix: Standards and Ethics of the National Association of Rehabilitation Professionals in the Private Sector

Preamble

NARPPS members recognize the uniqueness of the private rehabilitation field. The conduct of members of a professional organization must be ethical at all times. NARPPS recognize the free enterprise system and believes that fair competition encourages the development of quality services to both the client and the referral source.

Professional Conduct by Discipline

The member is obligated to maintain technical competency at such a level that the recipient receives the highest quality of services that the member's discipline is capable of offering. The implementation of a rehabilitation plan for a client is a multidisciplinary effort. NARPPS members will conduct themselves in interdisciplinary relationship in such a way as to facilitate the contribution of all specialists involved for maximum benefit of the recipient of services and to bring credit to each discipline.

Minimal Standards for Service Delivery

Standards shall apply to those persons who are providing the services.

The services and submission of reports shall be provided in a timely fashion and shall respond to the purpose of the referral and include recommendations, if appropriate. All reports shall reflect an objective, independent opinion based on factual determinations within the provider's area of expertise and discipline. The reports of service and findings shall be distributed to appropriate parties and in compliance with all applicable legal regulations.

The member shall render only those services that the member is competent and qualified to perform.

The member has an obligation to withdraw from a professional relationship if it is believed that the participation will result in violation of the ethical standards of his/her professional discipline.

There shall be a stated rationale for the provision of services to be rendered to the client in the form of an identified objective or purpose.

The member shall refuse to participate in practices which are inconsistent with the standards established by regulatory bodies regarding the delivery of services to clients.

Members will adhere to all tenets of confidentiality.

At the time of initial referral, the member has the responsibility for identifying to the referral source and to the client what services are to be provided and practices to be conducted. This shall include the identification, as well as the clarification, of services that are available by that member.

Professional Education, Training and Experience

NARPPS supports the principle of accreditation of member rehabilitation companies on a voluntary basis.

NARPPS considers the following standards to be the minimum requirements for a Professional Rehabilitation Practitioner:

A. *Professional Rehabilitation Practitioner*

1. Holder of a Master or Doctorate degree in health-support services from an accredited institution, plus one year of experience in vocational rehabilitation or physical rehabilitation. At least one year shall have been spent in the rehabilitation of disabling conditions and/or diseases; or
2. Holder of a Baccalaureate degree in health-support services from an accredited institution, plus two years of experience in vocational rehabilitation or physical rehabilitation. At least one year shall have been spent in the rehabilitation of disabling conditions and/or diseases; or
3. Diploma in Nursing from an accredited institution, plus a current R.N. license, plus three years of experience in physical rehabilitation or vocational rehabilitation. At least one year shall have been spent in the rehabilitation of disabling conditions and/or diseases; or
4. Holder of any Baccalaureate degree, other than listed in No. 2 above, from an accredited institution, plus three years experience in vocational rehabili-

tation. At least two years shall have been spent in the rehabilitation of disabling conditions and/or diseases; or

B. *Associate Rehabilitation Practitioner*
Holder of an Associate degree or high school diploma, plus continuing education and five years experience in vocational rehabilitation, including counseling, evaluation and direct case services. Three of the five years shall have been spent in the rehabilitation of disabling conditions and/or diseases.

C. *Rehabilitation Intern*
An individual who meets the minimum education requirements but does not meet the experimental requirements must be supervised by a professional rehabilitation practitioner. The intern shall provide the name of the professional rehabilitation practitioner under whose direct supervision he/she will work. The supervisor will function as the primary case manager.

Advocacy

Advocacy is a term used when referring to the act of pleading the cause or coming to the aid of another. NARPPS members respect the integrity and interest of the people and groups with whom they work. With regard to disabled persons, advocacy takes into account such issues as the legal rights of handicapped people to achieve integration into the social, cultural and economic life of the general community.

The role of NARPPS member as an advocate is to protest and promote the welfare of disabled persons to minimize control over circumstances that interfere with their obtaining vocational independence. When there is conflict of interest between the disabled client and the NARPPS member's employing party, the member must clarify the nature and direction of his/her loyalty and responsibilities and keep all parties informed of that commitment. NARPPS supports legislation that provides for services and care to the disabled.

Testimony

NARPPS recognizes that a rehabilitation professional has a responsibility when requested, to provide objective testimony.

Rehabilitation professionals provide services within the legal system and, in addition, to providing primary care rehabilitation services, are called upon to testify as to facts of which they have knowledge or to render a professional opinion on rehabilitation questions or disability factors affecting an individual.

The testimony of a rehabilitation professional should be limited to the specific fields of expertise of that individual as demonstrated by training, education and experience. The extent of the professional's training, education and experience needed to testify are determined by the legal jurisdiction in which the professional is testifying.

It is also permissible for a rehabilitation professional to render an expert opinion and answer questions about a disabled or handicapped individual that has been evaluated either in person or hypothetically.

Confidentiality

The purpose of confidentiality is to safeguard information that is obtained in the course of practice. Disclosures of information are restricted to what is necessary, relevant and verifiable with respect to the client's right to privacy. When a third party is involved, the key to confidentiality, when considering personal or confidential information, is to make certain that the client is aware, from the outset, that the delivery of services is being observed by the third party. Professional files, reports and records shall be maintained under conditions of security and provision will be made for their destruction when appropriate.

Business Practices

Individuals and/or organizations in private sector rehabilitation should adhere to all applicable standards and practices common to the general business community. In addition, they should give special attention to and adhere to the following specific points:

1. Members will adhere to all applicable federal, state and local laws establishing and regulating business practices.
2. Members will not misrepresent themselves, their duties or credentials.
3. Members should carry professional liability insurance for the protection of themselves and affected third parties.
4. Professional Rehabilitation Practitioners shall not engage in claims practices as such are defined under the statutes and legal precedents in their respective jurisdictions.
5. It is to be encouraged that any discussion and comments or criticism directed toward a fellow Professional Rehabilitation Practitioner or organization shall be positive and/or constructive.
6. Competitive advertising should be factually accurate and shall avoid exaggerated claims as to costs and results.
7. When asked to comment on cases being actively managed by another Professional Rehabilitation Practitioner organization, the reviewer shall make every reasonable effort to conduct an in-person evaluation before rendering his conclusion.
8. A rehabilitation practitioner member will not promise or offer services or results he cannot deliver or has reason to believe he cannot provide.
9. A member is not to solicit referrals either directly or indirectly by offering money or gifts other than the "de minimis" gifts to a referral source.
10. When recruiting an employee, members should not falsely promise benefits, employment advancement or salaries which they know or have reason to know they cannot meet.
11. No Rehabilitation Professional Practitioner or organization shall effectuate or participate in the wrongful removal of professional rehabilitation files or other materials upon the initiation of new employment.
12. Professional Rehabilitation Practitioners shall not enter into fee arrangements that would be likely to create conflicts of interest or influence their

testimony in claims cases. The Professional Rehabilitation Practitioners shall advise the referral source/payor of its fee structure in advance of the rendering of any services and shall also furnish, upon request, detailed accurate time records.

13. Member referral sources working for member organizations or individuals shall pay invoices in accordance with normal payment practices.

Peer Review

The function of the Peer Review Committee will be to investigate and rule on alleged infraction of the approved standards and ethics of NARPPS members. The Peer Review Committee will consist of the following:

a. Rehabilitation Counselor
b. Rehabilitation Nurse
c. Vocational Evaluator
d. Placement Specialist
e. Insurance Claimsperson or buyer
f. Private Practitioner (general)
g. Company administrator

References

American Personnel and Guidance Association. *Ethical standards casebook*. Washington, D.C.: APGA, 1976.

American Psychological Association. Revised ethical standards of psychologists. *APA Monitor*, 1977, *7*(3).

American Psychological Association (Division 22). Proposed platform. *Rehabilitation Psychology*, 1972, *19*(3), 142–143.

Bozarth, J. D. Philosophy and ethics in rehabilitation counseling. In R. M. Parker & C. E. Hansen (Eds.) *Rehabilitation Counseling*. Boston: Allyn and Bacon, Inc., 1981.

Brubaker, D. Professional status of rehabilitation counseling. In R. M. Parker & C. E. Hansen (Eds.), *Rehabilitation Counseling*. Boston: Allyn and Bacon, 1981.

Dellario, D. J. Rehabilitation research: A need for perspective. *Journal of Rehabilitation*, 1978, *44*(3), 137–139.

Deneen, L. J., & Hessellund, T. A. *Vocational rehabilitation of the injured worker*. San Francisco: Rehabilitation Publications, 1981.

Division of Industrial Accidents of the State of California. Rules and regulations of the administrative director, division of industrial accidents pertaining to rehabilitation. As amended 7/24/79.

Glaser, E. M. Ethical issues in consultation with organizations. *Consultation*, 1981, *1*(1), 12–16.

Keith, R. A. Physical rehabilitation: Is it ready for the revolution? *Rehabilitation Literature*, 1969, *30*, 170–173.

Lewin, S. S., Ramseur, J. H., & Sink, J. M. The role of private rehabilitation: Founder, catalyst, competitor. *Journal of Rehabilitation*, 1979, *45*(3), 16–19.

Lynch, R. K., & Martin, T. Rehabilitation counseling in the private sector: A training needs survey. *Journal of Rehabilitation*, 1982, *48*(3), 51–53, 73.

Matkin, R. E. The certification dilemma in private rehabilitation. *Journal of Applied Rehabilitation Counseling*, 1981, *12*(1).

McMahon, B. T. Private sector rehabilitation: Benefits, dangers and implications for educators. *Journal of Rehabilitation*, 1979, *45*(3), 56–58.

National Association of Rehabilitation Professionals in the Private Sector. *NARPPS standards and ethics*. Arcadia, Calif: NARPPS, 1981.

National Rehabilitation Counseling Association. Ethical standards for rehabilitation counseling. *Journal of Applied Rehabilitation Counseling*, 1972, *3*(4), 353–356.

Ross, E. M. Legislative trends in workers' compensation rehabilitation. *Journal of Rehabilitation*, 1979, *45*(3), 56–58.

Sanchez, I., Workman, E. L., Morris, G. M., Miller, J., & Edelstein, M. *The California workers' compensation rehabilitation system*. New York: MacMillan, 1981.

Scher, P. L. NARPPS — Key to the survival of rehabilitation in the nineteen-eighties. *Journal of Rehabilitation*, 1979, *45*(3), 50–51, 74.

Taylor, L. J. Toward a humanistic-existential rehabilitation psychology: A study of the congruence of the principles of rehabilitation psychology with the tenets of the humanistic-existential approach in psychology. Unpublished doctoral dissertation, University of Southern California, 1980.

Vocational Evaluation and Work Adjustment Association. Code of ethics. *VEWAA Bulletin*, 1971, *4*(3), 25–28.

Welch, G. T. The relationship of rehabilitation with industry. *Journal of Rehabilitation*, 1979, *45*(3), 30–31.

Wright, B. Value-laden beliefs and principles for rehabilitation psychology. *Rehabilitation Psychology*, 1972, *19*(1), 38–45.

14 Looking Ahead

Lewis J. Taylor, Gary Golter,
Marjorie Golter, and
Thomas E. Backer

The practice of vocational rehabilitation has gone through many changes in recent years. The major impetus for this change occurred in the mid-70s when rehabilitation services became a mandatory benefit in the California Workers' Compensation Act. Subsequently there was a proliferation of private vocational rehabilitation firms entering this new marketplace and offering their services directly to insurance carriers. The owners of these firms, most of whom were counselors by training, with the insurance carriers and the providers of supportive services, such as work evaluation, have created a new multimillion dollar industry that has been in flux since its conception.

The foundation of private rehabilitation is based upon identification and development of the strengths of the individual, not upon a preoccupation with weaknesses and problems. Private rehabilitation has grown in sophistication by focusing on transferable skills; support from the family, insurance carrier, and employer; job site modification; and other positive approaches. It has also diversified into other businesses such as consultation, computerization, and expert testimony. Out of this growth and movement certain problems, issues, and trends have emerged which will be the subject of our closing remarks. They include

- The cooperation between the public and private rehabilitation sectors;
- The interfacing between rehabilitation professionals and insurance personnel;
- The objectives of rehabilitation in the private sector;
- The difficulties for rehabilitation professionals in becoming business people;
- The ethical dilemmas of the private sector rehabilitation professional;
- Credentialing and training; and
- The fast-growing new areas of work in the rehabilitation field.

Cooperation between the Public and Private Sectors

For years the private and public sectors competed for business. Now it is becoming apparent that each has a place and that injured workers are best served by a cooperative effort. Since the private-for-profit rehabilitation company and the public vocational rehabilitation agency each have their strengths, to provide the best services to the disabled client there will need to be a collaboration of efforts. This collaboration could include a reciprocal referral process, cooperation in job placement, joint training programs, and mutual funding of rehabilitation service facilities. The future will call upon both the public and private sectors to integrate the best each has to offer in terms of service delivery, training, and referral distribution to guarantee quality rehabilitation services for the disabled client.

The challenge will be letting go of certain aspects of the job of rehabilitation as each sector becomes more aware and accepting of the other's expertise. If both sectors were not competing for the same business, more effort could be directed toward doing what each does best. The problem of competition and letting go of portions of the market will become more complicated with recent cutbacks in federal support for human services and the need of the public sector to become more "profitable" and "businesslike." The solution may evolve from the fact that since rehabilitation is an exceedingly difficult business both sectors will need all the help they can get in placing the injured worker. Also, as insurance carriers learn more about making referrals, the division of expertise may become more clearly defined. We can only speculate as to whether private and public sectors will choose to work together or will be forced into working together.

The Rehabilitation/Insurance Interface

Another issue that has evolved is the interface between rehabilitation practitioners and insurance personnel. It is the rehabilitation practitioner's responsibility not only to sell services to the insurance industry but also to establish a positive rapport with each referral source. In order to accomplish this successfully, the private sector practitioner must fully understand the insurance industry. All insurance companies are different; each has different goals, objectives, business mixes, and markets, and each services its product line differently. It is critical that private sector rehabilitation counselors understand these differences, speak the language of the customer (the insurance carrier), and most of all be responsive to the needs of the customer.

A problem that is beginning to emerge as rehabilitation counselors are trying to learn more about the insurance industry is that in trying to solicit business, they are complying more and more with insurance expectations. The question becomes: Is the injured worker receiving a nonbiased professional evaluation? Many practitioners experience being torn between the interests of the injured worker, the interests of the insurance company, and the interests of their employers. Knowledge of the insurance industry can be used merely to "market" or solicit business: "Tell me what you want, and I will give it to you." A better strategy would be: "Let me thoroughly understand my environment and, as a professional, I can best serve the injured worker."

Objectives of Rehabilitation

The objectives of rehabilitation in the private sector have become an issue because they are in some ways quite different from those of rehabilitation in the public sector.

Over the years there has been much discussion as to what services the private sector rehabilitation client is entitled to and what rehabilitation means when dealing with an injured worker. Can a plumber with a high-school education expect to be educated at the college level so that he can find work he is physically able to do? Most counselors have been trained with a "public-sector orientation" whereby education is a feasible and common means to the end, employment. However, since the majority of injured workers don't even have a high-school education, formal education cannot generally be used in their rehabilitation plans. As a consequence, a new concept has developed: the utilization of "transferable skills." The private sector rehabilitation practitioner now analyzes the pre-injury job in terms of what it took to do that job and assesses whether the injured worker has any skills that could be applied (transferred) to a new job. Using acquired skills has proven to be the most cost-effective means of returning the injured worker to gainful employment.

We might expect then that large employers will become more involved in the rehabilitation process with their own employees. To facilitate in-house rehabilitation, a company's job descriptions need to be precise and accurate, assistive devices need to be considered for the modification of preinjury jobs, and the personnel department needs to consider the hiring of their own injured workers before going outside to fill positions. As automation, cultural differences, and changes in the economy affect the requirements of jobs, industrialists and businessmen must understand that people can be utilized as they are and can be assisted to be productive in an ever-changing work setting. We may be seeing the need for a new education system for the express purpose of placing workers in jobs of the future. Control Data Corporation has addressed this issue with their computer-based PILOT System, used as part of their HOMEWORK Program to retrain injured employees to be computer programmers, many of them working from their own homes.

Rehabilitationists in Business

Another emerging issue is that of the rehabilitation professional as entrepreneur. The business of private rehabilitation has grown to be "big business" and needs to be managed well. Issues such as financial projections, planning, growth, and marketing are all part of the business. Is the rehabilitation professional trained to do that kind of work? Are we going to see rehabilitation firms of the future run by business people or owned by large insurance companies? The trend seems to be in that direction. IRA, Crawford, and Constitution Rehabilitation are all owned by insurance companies. The small rehabilitation practitioner has much to offer the field. A future concern will be how to ensure their survival.

Ethical Dilemmas

The ethical dilemmas facing the private sector practitioner involve changing roles. During the development of the private sector, the "client" identification has shifted from the worker to the bill payer. Therefore, the definition of rehabilitation has become less defined by the worker and counselor and more defined by the insurance carrier and employer. Counselors and owners of rehabilitation firms are constantly dealing with this dilemma and have yet to find an adequate answer.

In order for the private sector rehabilitation counselor to act positively in an environment containing potential professional conflict, it is imperative that the refinement of ethical standards be given a higher priority. Potential conflicts include but are not limited to the profit motive versus an orientation to human service delivery, competition between service providers, litigation, vested interests, and differing rehabilitation goals. Perhaps the managers of private sector rehabilitation firms will come together and form enforceable industry-wide policies that will help resolve the conflicts and dilemmas faced by the private sector practitioners. These industry leaders can help do the groundwork for dealing with the issues of rehabilitation goals, competition, unfair marketing practices, and other problems created by a rapidly growing and highly competitive service industry that significantly affects the lives of thousands of disabled persons.

Credentials and Training

The issue of credentials and training for rehabilitation professionals will need resolving in the future. The field has changed so drastically that there are very few schools that actually teach many of the jobs that are now done. Second, there are very few states where rehabilitation credentials hold any weight. (Minnesota, for example, requires a credential — the O.R.C. — to allow one to work with a client but this is unusual.)

The issue of training is resolving itself in two ways. One, the professors who teach rehabilitation counselors are becoming more aware of the private sector versus public-sector job duties and are making a distinction in the classroom. In addition, schools like Stout State University in Wisconsin are offering training specifically for private sector vocational rehabilitation counselors and are turning out counselors with job placement skills, *Dictionary of Occupational Titles* (D.O.T.) expertise, and evaluation knowledge. Secondly, the job of the vocational rehabilitation counselor is separate and distinct from that of the job placement specialist. As a matter of fact, the fourth edition supplement (1982) to the D.O.T. has a description of Job Development Specialist quite separate from Vocational Rehabilitation Counselor, each with unique job duties and qualifications. This separation has clarified the job duties, qualifications, and credentials for each and will continue in this direction in the future.

Expanding Professional Opportunities

The future will offer many exciting career options for private sector practitioners. In addition to the already diverse group of established occupations (counselor, job placement specialist, work evaluator, marketing representative, supervisor, and manager), new career choices continue to develop. For instance, the special knowledge and expertise of rehabilitation practitioners will be applied through private consultation to many settings. The development of a consulting practice requires a great deal of planning and assessment of one's special capabilities. Whether a consultant plans a practice around serving public sector agencies, the private sector, regulatory agencies, insurance companies, or self-insured employers, the opportunities for rehabilitation practitioners in organizational consulting should expand as practitioners become more adept at recognizing and marketing their unique capabilities to a marketplace that badly needs these specialized talents.

The increasing demand within the courts for expert witness testimony concerning a person's employability has also developed career opportunities for rehabilitation practitioners who wish to redirect their work toward the courtroom. Due to the qualifications required for a vocational expert, both formal and informal, and the difficulties inherent in testifying, it is obvious that expert testimony is not for everyone. However, with the trend toward increased litigation in personal injury claims, it would certainly appear that the role of the expert witness will be a growing specialty that will offer many personal challenges and satisfactions.

As employers begin to realize how the quality of employee assistance programs can be improved by offering employees help with career decisions and programs to reduce illnesses and work-related injuries, many career opportunities in this area will open in industry for rehabilitation practitioners. The cost-effectiveness of reducing employee turnover by improving the work environment and utilizing rehabilitation as a management tool to maximize the effectiveness of its work force supports the utilization of these programs. Once the experience of a few forward-looking companies, such as Control Data Corporation, 3M, and Sears, receive the proper exposure in personnel management circles, we can expect significant growth in this area of employment for rehabilitation practitioners.

The rehabilitation computer expert is another new career opportunity for rehabilitation practitioners and perhaps the most exciting to surface in several years. Currently there are a handful of counselors in the United States who have, mostly through chance, become technically competent as systems analysts or computer programmers. There is a critical need for the application of computer technology to the difficult tasks of selecting and locating new jobs for disabled workers. It is the technically trained counselor who will be called upon to deal with the issues of counselor-computer interface and to dissolve the remaining barriers to computer utilization so rehabilitation practitioners can take complete advantage of the computer revolution.

A broader issue is how rehabilitation counselors in the private sector will practice their profession in the future. What a counselor will do in the future is an issue in flux and involving all aspects of rehabilitation. If we were to write a job description for a counselor today and for one five years from now, the job descriptions would be vastly different. First of all, in the future counselors will be more aware of the "data" part of their job. They will be using computers in many different ways to make their work more efficient. It will be crucial for them to understand what it takes to play various rehabilitation roles. Training for counselors will need to develop from using only a "mini-therapist" orientation to include a job specialist and placement orientation. It appears that over the years we will see a distinct change in the job descriptions of counselors who work in public and private settings. Perhaps a collaboration of the two will result from the reliance one has on the other in performing different services for disabled people—workers and nonworkers.

Today these new career fields are related only tangentially to the private rehabilitation industry. How rapidly they will grow and become formalized is yet to be seen. The public agency uses consultation on a national basis far more than the private sector does. However, companies are starting to develop to sell computer technology and services specially to private sector rehabilitation companies. Some rehabilitation companies are diversifying into these new market areas as a hedge against a changing and fickle workers' compensation market. The owners of these firms are finding that running a large service organization is a tedious and arduous task and that market diversification adds excitement and change of pace to their jobs. In addition, there are difficult and unique problems associated with marketing rehabilitation services to be solved. Maybe the future will see a separate marketing organization selling the rehabilitation services of several firms with rehabilitation companies becoming more specialized as the years go by. It is clear that there is plenty of business to go around, and perhaps specialization will be a trend of the future, allowing room for public and private agencies, large national companies, small statewide companies, and individual counselors acting as sole proprietors. The first and foremost concern must be with the injured worker and the service he or she is entitled to and will receive as the field grows and changes.

In conclusion, the future looks very exciting for rehabilitation practitioners in the private sector. Expanding and diversified career opportunities, better working relationships with the public sector, a more professional work environment, and an expanding marketplace are just some of the positive trends in private sector rehabilitation today.

Index

Index